Mssiee Lyn -
Let's pray
for a cure -
Kathy

My Mother
Is Losing
Her Memory

and

I Am Losing

My Mind

Parenting the Aging Parent

Kathleen Bjork

BirchTree Publications Copyright © 2017 by Kathleen Bjork
Palm Desert, CA

ISBN **978-0-9990369-0-7**

Front cover: Dunn & Associates

10 9 8 7 6 5 4 3 2 1

In Memorium
with love
to

My Mother

Forward

Do you have a parent who can't perform many tasks they easily used to do? Is your mother or father requiring more of your help? You are not alone. My mother was in her late eighties when I began to notice that she had problems remembering, and for the next ten years I watched a steady decline in her abilities. It is hard to watch a vibrant, capable person undergo changes that they struggle with and may deny.

Thanks to the advancement in medicine, more people like my mother are living longer healthier lives. Those in my generation who are into our sixties and seventies have raised our children and are ready to enjoy retirement. However, we are sometimes faced with caring for an aging parent. This parent may have physical health problems, but the ones most vexing are the mental ones.

We hear a lot about Alzheimer's disease and sometimes joke about it when we have a "senior moment," but we know the reality of it is tragic. Oftentimes, we hear about someone with the extreme symptoms of Alzheimer's where the person doesn't recognize his loved ones and becomes almost catatonic. In reality, the progression of dementia differs with each person and with each type, with Alzheimer's being just one kind. That said, there is a common pattern to dementia which carries no cultural or geographic boundaries. When I began this journey with my mother I had just a general idea of what dementia was, and it was only after I had been taking care of her for a while that I looked up the symtoms. I was able to check off almost every one.

It was only after relating my many stories about difficulties with my mother to friends, and hearing stories about problems with their aging parents that I decided to share my story. Believe me, I don't have all the answers. However, if sharing my experiences of my mother's journey into dementia can help someone else realize that the challenges and struggles they face in caring for a loved one with dementia are not unique, I will have met my goal.

This is my mother's experience and my story.

Kathy Bjork

October 2017

There is a moral task of caregiving, and that involves just being there, being with that person and being committed. When there is nothing that can be done, we have to be able to say, "Look, I'm with you in this experience. Right through to the end of it."

Dr. Arthur Kleinman

Prologue

This is the story of my mother and her experience with dementia, but the beginning lies much earlier. It begins with my grandmother.

It was in the Spring of 1961. Eighteen and a freshman in college, I was still living at home with my parents when my grandparents drove down from their cabin in Blue Jay for a visit one morning. Only it wasn't just a *visit*. My mother had other plans—ones that would change my grandmother's life forever.

In the last few weeks, my mother had been in communication with her Uncle Edgar, Grandma's younger brother. Mom said Grandma had become paranoid and hallucinated. She threatened my grandfather, once with a knife, and she was afraid what Grandma would do. Edgar helped her work out a solution; he would be meeting her that morning. I did know Grandma had problems with depression, and had undergone electric shock treatments several times in her life, but I never saw this side of her.

My grandparents were both a special part of my life. They lived in Riverside for as long as I could remember. When Daddy was away during the war my mother and sister and I lived with them. They had only recently moved from their large two story house when it had to be sold and demolished to build the Riverside 91 freeway.

Grandma doted on my sister and me. She was very creative and often made us things. I still have the life-size doll she made for me when I was seven, along with a pine needle basket and several quilts.

The last image I have of my grandmother that morning she was standing in the kitchen. She was getting a glass of cold water from the refrigerator, talking to me and laughing. I don't know what excuse my mother gave her, but later that morning she left with her. I wished them goodbye. First, I wanted to run after them yelling, "Stop!" Then I wanted to cry.

I was not in the courtroom, but I could imagine what happened that day when the judge declared Grandma incompetent and she was taken away to Patton Mental Hospital. She probably cried, yelled and even screamed at my mother. I would have. It was a betrayal. I never knew what actually took place, because Mom never talked about it and we somehow knew not to ask.

Over the next several months, I went with my mother on visits to Patton to see Grandma. She had a small, cold, private room, but most of the time we saw her in the large open area with all the other patients. On my first visit I saw a completely different person. My happy, always neatly-dressed grandmother wore a housecoat with a blanket wrapped around her shoulders, and was very subdued. She was glad to see us, but confused. I looked around the room. She doesn't belong here, I thought. She's my grandma who always loved me, not like these other people.

The residents in the room were involved in a myriad of activities, and different scenarios were taking place. Some were pacing back and forth talking to themselves, while others were curled up next to a wall or in a chair with a vacant expression on their faces. A man was yelling at an imaginary person, while a woman was gently soothing her baby doll. There were about fifty people sitting or milling around the room, and a constant undercurrent of talking was present while we tried to visit.

We would bring pudding or Jello for her to eat, Mom spooning it into her mouth. As we continued going to see her, she became more confused and thought Grandpa was with her, but in the other room. Mom became younger to her, and when my sister went to see her, she thought my sister was my mother. After a while, her physical health began to deteriorate also. When we came, we had to clean the pus that seeped out of the bottom of her feet. Mom said it was the result of heart disease and the accumulation of fluids that were being released from her body.

Mom had been in contact with the director of the hospital trying to get help for Grandma throughout her stay, but the staff was ill-equipped to handle that many patients, and were prone to administer medicine to subdue, rather than provide needed counseling. After days of phone calls, the director finally admitted her to the hospital unit, but by then it was too late. The last time I saw Grandma she lay in an adult-size crib with very high sides. She died a week later.

Mom never talked about this time, but for several years, every Christmas, we wrapped presents such as socks, housecoats, and snacks, and took them to Patton Hospital for the patients. Mom also began seeing a counselor.

As a eighteen-year-old, this experience affected me profoundly, enough so that I changed my major to psychology. With age, I overcame the resentment I felt for what my mother had done, and understood the emotional toll it must have taken on her. In the 1960s society did not recognize dementia as we do now. Those who acted out or were uncontrollable were treated as mentally ill and hospitals were filled with the elderly, like my grandmother. I now realize, faced with few options, my mother was only doing the best she could at the time.

I have often thought about my grandmother over the years, but never more so than when I became the caregiver daughter, and faced the enormous respon-siblities and decisions, especially the difficult ones, that needed to be made for my mother.

Alone

Daddy died at eighty-one. He had been diagnosed with colon cancer two years earlier. That was the year we took our last camping trip with him to June Lake in the Sierras. He loved the mountains and hiking the John Muir trails, and would tell everyone about the time he hiked to the top of Mount Whitney, the highest peak in California. My family often went camping near Mammoth in the summers when I was a child, and my husband and I continued the tradition with our own two children. This time, my kids were living on their own, so my young nephews went with us.

Two weeks after we returned, Dad had his operation. My sister, Barb, and I were sitting in the waiting room with my mother when the doctor came out to talk with her. We had hoped for the best, but the news wasn't good. "We got all the cancer from his colon," he said, "but found numerous tumors throughout his abdomen." In other words, the cancer had metastasized into the rest of his body. So began his endless periods of chemotherapy.

Daddy never let the disease or treatment depress him, or at least, he didn't show it. He got up and dressed every day and took his three mile walks as long as he was able. As I look back, I admire his courage. Up until the end, when his stomach blew up to the size of a beach ball and the cancer was pressing down on his organs, I never heard him complain.

Mom was remarkable at this time too, showing patience and perseverance. She was his sole caregiver taking him to all his appointments, making sure he ate well and took his medications. His last two years were a mellow time in my parents' relationship. I think knowing they didn't have much time left, they grew closer. Mom once told me when Daddy couldn't sleep at night they would lie in bed and talk about the past.

Mom and Dad were married for fifty-eight years, but they had known each other for sixty-nine. They met in seventh grade, were a couple all through high school, and married when she was twenty-two and he twenty-three. They were together all that time except when he left for Europe in 1943 during the war.

After Daddy died, Mom carried on her usual activities which helped fill the void left in her life. She went to church on Sundays, volunteered at the community hospital two days a week, played bridge with her girlfriends, and went to lunch with friends a couple of times a month. My brother, sister, and I tried to visit as much as we could, and she also came to visit us.

What was difficult were the nights. She avoided going to bed. Always a night-owl, she now often fell asleep sitting up in a chair in the living room. I'm sure lying in bed awake and alone was something she feared. After a while, she developed swelling in her legs and per doctor's instructions we put a board under her mattress to raise her legs to help circulation. She also began to sleep with a heating pad to ease her arthritis.

Over the next few years she stayed in good health except for the arthritis. She received shots in her spine to relieve sciatica pain, but it only helped a little. Her toes were now curled up so she had to put her high heels away and mostly wear canvas shoes. Doug and Barb both lived in Arizona, but it was only an hour and a half drive for me so I was the one to see her more often.

After I retired, I made sure to go with her to her doctor appointments. I wanted to keep apprised of what the doctor said, since I couldn't always rely on Mom's memory and she would downplay her ailments or not tell the doctor everything he should know. After her appointments, we'd eat at her favorite restaurant, Marie Callender's, and then go shopping at CVS pharmacy and Trader Joe's which were across the street from the restaurant. She always made a list of what she needed. At this time she was still able to walk on her own, but I noticed at home she'd grab onto the furniture as she made her way around the house. When we pulled up to CVS I would get out first to find a basket, then roll it back to the car for Mom. It kept her stable as she wheeled around the store. She needed a walker, but whenever someone suggested it, she dug in her heels and insisted she didn't need one.

Mom didn't go to college, but she was smart and would've done well because she had a good memory. She was in her late eighties when we began to see changes. She would forget where she put things and repeat something she had previously said. We especially noticed it in phone conversations. At first, I attributed it to the fact that Mom's world was getting smaller as she lost friends and didn't go out as often. Then I came to realize it was her memory. She really did not know she had already told me something. She'd tell me about her sink being fixed or the latest story of what someone did or didn't do, and then I'd hear it all over again the next week when I called. I knew she couldn't help it, so at first I'd politely listen. After a while I learned to steer the conversation to another topic or find something to do while she was talking, carrying the phone with me.

When we were with her, she was capable of carrying on a conversation, but sometimes asked the same question again and again. When she mixed up her facts, I tried to gently correct her, but after awhile I just let it go to save an argument.

Observing these changes I didn't need a doctor's opinion to know Mom was in the beginning stages of dementia.

The Check's in the Mail

Mom never talked to us about her finances. She wouldn't even tell us how much Daddy earned or the amount of her pension check. She prided herself on being self reliant and wouldn't think of asking for help. But the day finally came when I knew I needed to step in and offer assistance.

I started to pay close attention when she talked about the bills she needed to pay. She told me that several times Verizon or the gas or electric company called about her bill, and she paid over the phone using her debit card. She just laughed it off, but I worried that someday she wouldn't pay in time and be left in the dark or with her phone cut off and us unable to reach her.

One time when I spoke with her she said she was writing checks that day. I could picture her sitting at the kitchen table with the bills spread out before her as she always did.

I called her a few days later.

"How are you, Mom?" I asked

" Oh, I'm fine," she replied. I was supposed to go to lunch with Betty Jane, but her back started bothering her. You know she has that problem and she's not getting any better . . . "

"Say Mom, the other day you were working on your bills. Were you able to finish and get them mailed?"

"Oh no," she said, with a sigh. "They make them so hard to understand now. They're still sitting on the table. I'd better pay them or they'll be calling me again."

I knew I needed to do something. This was getting serious.

My mother was always very independent, even when my father was alive. She had definite ideas about the way things should be done and was extremely organized. In contrast to my sporadic record keeping, she kept a balanced checkbook and a journal where she wrote everything she spent each month. She liked to boast that she had journals for every year since she married, fifty-nine in all.

The next week when I visited I went in the den and found her latest journal. As I began skimming through, I saw her last entries were in sharp contrast to her earlier ones. My mother's usual neat, precise handwriting was light and shaky. She had gotten mixed up on some of the months and even wrote the wrong year a few times. I knew I needed to help her, but I'd have to proceed slowly.

I walked into the kitchen where she was sitting. "Mom, you know how you have been having problems with your bills. Why don't you let me do them for you?"

She reacted as I knew she would. "I have been paying my bills all my life, I don't need any help."

"Paying my bills is really easy," I explained. "The phone and the electric company bills are paid automatically. The amount I owe is taken right from my bank account."

"I don't know. I like to keep track of my account."

"You will still get your monthly statement. I can look up your account on my computer. I pay all my bills online on my computer."

After I convinced her that this way she wouldn't have to worry about missing payments or her phone or electricity shut off, she finally agreed.

I took her bills home with me, but what seemed like an easy job to set up payments, turned out to take hours of phone calls, computer time and paperwork.

I was put on hold and they refused to talk to me unless my mother was on the line. Half of her accounts were still in my father's name. They didn't know that he had been gone for twelve years. I had to create numerous account passwords for websites, give out personal information, and was required to mail numerous 'Power of Attorneys'. My mother's Social Security number? I had it memorized. What I learned, though–sometimes it's much easier to just pretend to be my mother.

Luckily, we had visited her lawyer and had a trust drawn up a few years earlier which gave me Power of Attorney and allowed me to handle her money. I gradually took over all of her banking and had sole use of her ATM card to deposit and withdraw any money she needed. She was mad about it, although she didn't complain to me. She did bemoan to my brother and sister, "Kathy tries to control me. I can take care of my own money. I have been paying bills for years!"

She continued to gripe about needing money, but she couldn't keep track of it. She had two small coin purses as well as her wallet and glasses case in her purse, and money could be found in any one of them. She also sometimes hid money in her nightstand drawer and forgot she put it there. Her checkbook was a mess which I allowed her to keep so she would feel she had some control.

It was a decision I would later regret.

There's Nothing Wrong with My Driving

Unlike Europeans with their extensive rail and bus systems, we Americans rely on our cars, which become almost extensions of ourselves. With its multitude of freeways and suburbs, this is even more so in Southern California. If you take a Californian's car away, it is almost like sealing them off from the outside world. So it was for my extremely independent mother. If she needed something from the store, she was there in just minutes. She drove to church on Sundays and met friends for lunch, although as the years went by lunch dates were fewer as her friends could no longer meet. " All my friends are dead or are incapacitated and can't get out any more," she would lament. "If my car were taken away from me, I think I would kill myself." She felt that strongly about it, so we knew when the time came we'd be faced with resistance.

For several years my sister tried to talk with her about her driving, and Mom would become indignant that Barb would even suggest that she not drive anymore. I agreed with my sister, but avoided discussing it with Mom. However, I did notice her reactions were slower and she got mixed up when she drove somewhere not on her regular routes. The summer she turned eighty-nine, and talked about having the great grandchildren visit and driving them to the beach, we cringed.

Later that year when she drove seventy miles to our house for Thanksgiving, she told us a story about the "awful driver who suddenly stopped right in front of me on the freeway on ramp." The bumper on her Honda was caved in and part of the hood raised. She also had another accident we learned about later, one she neglected to tell us. I only found out about this encounter when her hairdresser called me because she was concerned and thought the family should know.

"One evening," she related, "your mother drove to CVS pharmacy to pick up her prescriptions. When she pulled into a parking place her car kept going and it ran into some bushes. The car's front bumper and hood were damaged and she had it repaired. She didn't want you to know."

Of course we wanted to know. My mother could be very clever when it suited her purpose. How could she continue to say she had no accidents and that she was a good driver if we knew what she had done?

The deciding moment came when she drove 320 miles to visit my sister in Yuma, Arizona. I was out all day, but home in the evening when my sister called.

"Have you heard from Mom?" she asked.

Mom had started out that morning and ran into some "car trouble" along the way. She told my sister she wasn't sure she would be able to continue, and she might have to call me for help because she was closer to Palm Desert than Yuma. I did not have my cell phone with me that morning and was not aware of any missed calls.

Just as I yelled to my husband in the next room to check for messages on my cell phone, Barb said, "Oh good, Mom just drove up." Before I had time to even react to her comment, she exclaimed, "Oh no, she just ran into the house!"

An hour later my sister called back.

My mother had indeed pulled into their graveled driveway and run into their carport. She was okay, but she easily could have hit her fifteen-year-old great grandson who had opened the driveway gate for her.

"She ran into two pillars, knocked them completely off their foundations," Barb said.

"Oh my God! Where is the car? What did Mom say?"

"We called AAA and they towed it away. Mom's fine and she acts like it's no big deal. She's trying to play it down."

"Are you going to let her have the car back?"

"NO."

"I agree," I said. "This would be the perfect time to take it away"

When Barb explained to my mother that if she continued driving she might cause an accident and hurt herself or a child, it fell on deaf ears. I discovered that you can't reason with someone with dementia. Trying to talk to them is like trying to talk to a three year old. The car never came back to my mother from the repair shop. Barb and her husband Roy drove her back home. My brother and nephew picked up the car the next week and drove it to their house in Phoenix.

My mother was furious that her car "was taken away" from her. She would tell her tale of woe about how horrible her children were treating her to anyone who would listen.

She would tell us, her family, "My friends think it's just terrible the way you treat me. I can drive just fine. I don't need you to decide what I can and can't do!"

I had sympathy for Mom. I'd hate to not be able to drive, and if my car were taken away, I would be angry also. I hoped she would adjust and come to accept it, but I had my doubts. What bothered me most was how she complained to other people about us. Friends told us what she said. She twisted the facts around portraying herself as the innocent victim and us as the cold, heartless children.

Let Your Mother Live in the Comfort of Her Own Home

My mother's arthritis continued to worsen. She found it difficult to go into the yard to water her plants or do other simple tasks, yet she still insisted she could live on her own. One day she put soup on the stove and forgot about it. The house filled with smoke and the smoke alarm went off summoning several concerned neighbors. My brother, sister and I knew we were coming close to having "the talk." She could not live by herself anymore; she needed someone to help her.

I was encouraged when I took her for a doctor's appointment. When he noticed she had difficulty walking and she asked him the same questions over and over again, he realized how much worse she had become both mentally and physically.

He told her, "You should not be living by yourself. They have places now that are almost like a hotel. You can have your own room and they serve all your meals. I know a lot of people, like my father-in-law, who moved into assisted living and like it."

I should have known it would not convince my mother.

"Why should I go to someplace like that when I have my own home," she said as we were driving home.

She probably did feel like she had things under control. A gardener cut the grass and trimmed the bushes every week. Michele, the next-door neighbor, watered the plants in the yard, and a woman came every two weeks and cleaned her house. Since Doug removed the knobs from the stovetop and turned off the gas after the kitchen fire, she began to cook TV dinners every night in the microwave.

After she lost her car and couldn't drive, she required even more assistance. Even though Barb and I had our own families and activities we were involved in, we had no choice but to help. Every few weeks my sister or I visited to check on her and see if she needed anything. Though we stocked up on food, she missed being able to buy the fresh fruits and vegetables she loved. We especially worried about her eating TV dinners because of all the salt they contained. She was supposed to avoid salt because of the edema in her legs from sitting too much.

It was a long drive to Riverside for my sister, so I usually went to see Mom. Though retired, I was almost busier than when I had worked. More than begrudge the fact that I had to drive up to help her, I felt guilty when a week or two went by and I hadn't gone. "Go see Mom," was continually on my mental list of "to do" tasks. Mom had guilt feelings, also. When I did go see her, she apologized for needing my help. "You are so busy, I hate to have you spend your time helping me." Of course I assured her it was no problem at all.

Despite our efforts, we knew it wasn't enough. Someone needed to check on her on a regular basis. She was getting more forgetful and we were afraid someday she'd fall and fracture something. We were going to have to hire some help, someone to look in on her and take her to the store or shop for her.

So I made it my mission to thoroughly research senior home care agencies in the Riverside area. I phoned the County Senior Health Department for recommendations along with checking out places online. I narrowed it down to five, then called each agency and personally spoke with the director. I took copious notes. I wanted to choose the best one. Finally, I decided on one that seemed professional and caring. Their caregivers had ongoing training and kept daily logs when at a client's home. I made an appointment with Home Instead and arranged to be there when the woman from the agency came to talk with my mother.

The day she stopped by and explained what the agency could do for her, my mother seemed agreeable. The next day I talked with the woman and she felt it went well; she had worked out a schedule and they were set to start the next week.

The following Monday morning a caregiver from Home Instead arrived at the door. Mom refused to let her in. "I don't need any help," my mother informed her. They tried again the next day, and the next, with the same result. She sent them away. Finally, the agency director called me. "We can do nothing further. Your mother says she doesn't need help, and if she won't cooperate, we can't help."

Given time, we thought Mom would see that she needed help. It didn't happen. She became intent on showing us she could take care of herself. Instead of asking us for assistance, she called a neighbor or the one friend who still drove, and asked them to pick up things for her at the store or the pharmacy. Her hairdresser even drove her home from her hair appointments. These same people, who knew my mother's condition and told us she should not be living on her own, said they helped because they felt sorry for her. She also worked on their sympathy by complaining about us. We were so awful. We took her car away from her. "They just snatched my keys away from me," she would tell them. We were trying to control her life.

After a few months I tried another agency with the same outcome as the first one. Desperate, I tried a different approach. I told Mom we were hiring someone to drive her on errands. She could ask for their help only if she wanted; she was in control. This worked for a while. While we envisioned a schedule of prearranged times when she would be picked up to go to the store or to the hairdresser, Mom had a different plan. If she needed someone to drive her somewhere she called shortly before she wanted to go and expected them to come right away, like a taxi. Sometimes when they came for scheduled appointments, she canceled or wasn't ready when they arrived. She did not seem to understand that the agency hired people ahead-of-time based on the needs of clients. The caregivers had specific hours, and the agency liked the same caregiver to work with the client every time, if possible. My mother turned the whole system on its head.

One night I tried to call Mom. Receiving no answer on either her land line or her cell phone, I called the agency to check on her, as well as the neighbor across the street who had a key to the house. When she answered the door she didn't understand what the fuss was all about. She was just fine. Her cell phone had not been charged and her landline phone was off the hook.

We had nagged my mother many times to keep her cell phone charged. I also repeatedly pled with her to use the lifeline emergency system I had bought for her. I gave her the lanyard for her to wear around her neck. That is the last time I saw it on her. When asked why she didn't use it, she'd reply, " I don't need it; I can use my phone."

We Told You So

Early one morning I was sitting at the kitchen table reading the paper when the phone rang. It was my mother's minister. This took me by surprise. I knew Chris. He had officiated at my father's funeral several years earlier, but he had never called me before. I didn't know he had my phone number.

At first I couldn't understand what he was talking about. He was at my mother's house.

"I've tried to reach her by phone and get no answer," he explained. "She's probably lying on the floor hurt. Do you want me to break down the door or call 911?"

I was totally confused, but thought there was time for questions later. The top priority was to find out if my mother was all right.

"Break down the door if you have to," I told him, "then call 911 if you think she needs help."

I spent an anxious hour before he called back from the hospital emergency room. She had indeed fallen and was lying on the kitchen floor and couldn't get to the phone. He said she had lain there all night. A neighbor, and fellow church member, had stopped by and talked with my mother the evening before. She came in the back door and noticed my mother sitting on the floor next to the refrigerator and asked if she needed any help. My mother told her no, she had just dropped something, so she left. The next morning when the neighbor got no answer on the phone she alerted the minister.

Chris had carried her out to the car and driven her to the hospital himself. She didn't seem to be in much pain, and he and I concluded that it probably wasn't anything serious. He volunteered to stay with her until she was released. I considered driving to Riverside, but was reluctant to leave. My pregnant daughter was due to have our grandson induced the next morning, and we had volunteered to stay with our two year old granddaughter.

It was afternoon when I got the third call. They had taken X-rays and my mother had broken her hip. A surgeon had been contacted, and they were in the process of obtaining a hospital room for her. I felt rather embarrassed that the minister had stayed with her all that time through the many the examinations and procedures, but he assured me it was okay. I knew then I would have to make the ninety mile drive from Palm Desert to see her. I told him I would be coming and thanked him profusely for his help.

I left shortly thereafter and arrived at Riverside Community Hospital early evening. My mother was settled in her room, and as I was talking with her the surgeon came in. He explained to us exactly where the hip bone was broken and said they had scheduled surgery for the following day.

After the doctor left I pulled up a chair next to Mom's bed. "Are you in any pain?" I asked.

" A little," Mom answered. "But they have me all doped up with medicine, so I don't notice it much."

"What caused you to fall?"

"I was getting a TV dinner out of the freezer and when I closed the door and turned around to set it on the counter, I twisted my leg. When I tried to catch myself, I fell."

" So," I said. "you were on the floor <u>all night</u> and hadn't even eaten dinner?"

"Yes, but I didn't hurt too badly. Except every time I tried to scoot across the floor to reach the phone, I got sharp pains in my right leg ."

"And Evelyn came by. Why didn't you tell her you needed help?"

"Oh, I didn't want to bother her. And you know Evelyn. She's such a busybody, by the time she finished telling everyone the whole church would know." So much for pride, I thought.

"I could say something about your lifeline device <u>that you don't use,</u> but I won't," I said, shaking my head. She didn't react, and I decided that she didn't need a lecture right now.

"Remember, Ricki is going to have the baby induced tomorrow. We're taking care of Jayden."

She broke into a smile. "That's wonderful! How is she feeling?"

"She's fine. Just glad to finally get it over with."

"You shouldn't be here with me. You can leave. I'll be okay."

"No, I'm staying overnight at your house, of course. Doug is driving over early tomorrow. He said he'd call and talk to you tonight." Thankfully, Doug, my younger brother, would be here during her operation.

"I'm sorry to be such a bother," she said.

"Don't be silly," I answered. "You'd do the same for us."

I stayed and visited with my mother that evening and left early the next morning. I wish I could say that my mother changed her ways and learned from this painful lesson, but her strong determination to be independent kept that from happening.

Rehab Nightmares

My mother came through her hip operation just fine. For a ninety-two year old she did very well. A few years ago they probably would not have opted to operate on anyone that age.

As it turned out, our daughter delivered our grandson at the same time my mother was undergoing her operation.

Mom remained in the hospital for five days before she was released. After that her doctors called for her to stay at a nursing/rehabilitation center for a few months for extra care and physical therapy. Since I would have the responsibility to check on her and visit, we decided to have her stay at a rehab center in Palm Desert to save me all that driving. It would also be an hour and a half drive closer for my sister and brother. So Mom was transported ninety minutes by ambulance to a rehab hospital only five miles from my home.

My husband and I were there the evening the ambulance pulled up to the care facility. She seemed a little confused, but considering it was an unfamiliar place in a different city, it was understandable. The next morning I realized how mixed-up she really was. At 1 a.m. the phone rang. I groggily answered. It was my mother.

"Are you coming to get me?"

"What do you mean? You're in the hospital, Mom."

"I know. But I'm out in front waiting for you."

"You hurt your hip, Mom. You're supposed to stay in bed."

"No, I'm at the YMCA and need to get home."

The Y? Really? I thought.

Of course, I pictured my mother dragging herself out of bed, down the hall and flinging herself out the door onto the front sidewalk. But I knew this was an impossibility, so I called the nurses' station and asked them to please check on her. They called back half an hour later.

"Your mother is in bed and she is okay. I think she is hallucinating. We have put a band on her arm so if she does try to get out of bed it will sound an alarm."

This was just the first of many strange conversations we had with my mother over the next few weeks. She told us there was a basement in the building and the staff took her there for tests. (There is no basement) People were out to get her. She claimed the nurses' aides that helped her take a shower were Marines. (Wow!) She called friends and they called us. They were worried about her. What we did not know then, but learned later, was that people her age

27

sometimes have problems with the anesthesia and may exhibit bizarre behavior and hallucinations for a time afterward. Mom was a classic case.

She did finally begin to get back her sanity and start physical therapy. I tried to visit her every day and most of the time I found her in bed. I would look at her daily schedule.

" Why didn't you go to your therapy session this morning?" I would ask.

"I was too tired. " became her mantra.

I knew this was hard on her. My mother was not an exerciser. She never liked to even take a walk around the block at home, but if she wanted to get better and leave the rehabilitation hospital she needed to make the effort and cooperate with the physical therapist. It was exasperating. I felt like a mother trying to coax a child to do something that they didn't want to do, but needed to do for their own good.

I couldn't bribe her with lollipops so I began to schedule my visits right before her therapy session to make sure she followed through. When I arrived she was usually still in bed, but with the help of the aide we got her up and ready for her session. At first she was wheeled down to the PT room and back, but after awhile, as she improved, the physical therapist and I would slowly walk with her as she used her walker; when she grew tired the wheelchair was available for the rest of the way. Though Mom made more of an effort, she still had days when she didn't want to move, and when she was forced to walk it wasn't without some grousing.

I Thought You Cared

My family has always stayed close over the years, and my mother worked hard to see that it remained so. We celebrated most holidays together and she called us regularly. If she heard a family member was sick, she always called to see how they were doing. Though not an affectionate mother, she was concerned for our welfare and expressed her love by doing things for us. She was an excellent "nurse" when we were sick, and cared for me through many ear aches, the chicken pox, and measles.

It was while my mother was recuperating in the rehabilitation hospital that a routine visit for a mammogram disclosed some disturbing news. I was diagnosed with breast cancer. Though in shock for a few days–you immediately think of death–I came to accept it and put my faith in the doctors. I am not the type to worry, and I did not waste time dwelling on it; I would take it one day at a time. It was my reality–the cancer phase of my life. Even though the cancer was fast-growing, it was still in stage II. I did not keep the news private. I let my friends and relatives know, and asked them to send positive thoughts my way. With their support I would "get through."

What I was concerned about, however, was when to tell my mother. Though she was better, she still had her memory problems. I didn't know how she would react and didn't want to cause any setbacks or additional anguish. I finally decided to tell her, and to my surprise, it was me, not her, that it affected.

My mother was in bed that day when I entered her room. I asked her how she was, gave her some magazines I'd brought, and then prepared myself.

"Mom, I have breast cancer," I said.

I got a blank look.

"Mom," I said. "I have cancer. Remember, Daddy had cancer and you took care of him until he died."

"Oh. I thought your father died of a heart attack."

"No, he didn't. He had *cancer*, like I do."

With this, I started to cry. It took me by surprise. I thought I was brave and able to accept my diagnosis. But this was my mother. Intellectually, I knew she was not able to think rationally and was not completely in touch with reality, but emotionally I was still that little girl who wanted her mother to care.

Two months later, I had a mastectomy, followed by four months of chemotherapy and two months of radiation. In the months that followed I still talked about my cancer with my mother. I would tell her why I couldn't come to see her and explain my treatments.

Whether she ever truly understood, I don't know, but I think I needed to talk about it for me.

Assisted Living: The Big Decision

It finally came time to move Mom from her rehab facility. She wasn't leaving because she had reached her goals for physical therapy. Although she was walking with the walker on her own, she was still afraid, and her steps were more like shuffles. No, it was about money; Medicare would no longer pay for her care. After seeing her reports every month, I knew the hospital had done their best to extend her stay. She had simply used up the time allotted for someone to recover from her type of surgery. It had been three months.

Now she had to move somewhere, and it couldn't be back home. Because I would be having surgery, followed by chemotherapy treatments, I knew I could not drive to Riverside and check on her as I had in the past. So my siblings and I agreed that this would be the perfect time to have her move into an assisted living facility.

We decided it should be in Palm Desert. First, it was closer to Riverside and her home. Second, I was the logical choice to check on her on a regular basis. My younger brother, Doug, still worked and traveled out of town with his sales job, and Barb and Mom did not always get along. Though she was as concerned about

Mom as much as I was, when Mom became upset or said something negative, it was hard for my sister to remain calm. She would try to talk to Mom, she'd resist, then Barb would get angry or walk away in a huff. In cases like this, I usually "let it go" or tried to work around it.

The year before, when we considered moving Mom out of her home, I had checked out all the facilities in Palm Desert that were close to me with the aid of a Senior Living Options representative, who was of invaluable help. At that time, I had chosen a home that I thought would be a good fit for her. Each facility, I found, has its own personality. Some are very low-key and the residents are mellow and not very active. Others are extremely active, with residents out of their rooms and participating in a lot of activities. Others are a blend of the two. The age of residents is a key factor in the placement decision. Someone like my mother, who was in her nineties, would not fit in if the majority of residents were seventy- and early eighty-year-olds. She also would dislike a facility like one I visited where the residents sat around in a circle in their wheelchairs, no one talking or interacting.

The facility I liked, Legend Gardens, had a series of thirty-five apartments, each with their own living room, large bedroom, and handicap-equipped bathroom. The grounds were well manicured and it had a beautiful rose garden which I thought Mom would like. My sister and niece went with me to check them out once more. I made a deposit on a unit, and we were ready to move Mom in.

However, after conferring with her doctor and the nurses who had been taking care of her, we began to have second thoughts. They felt she needed to be where she could have more care. At Legend Gardens she would be living more independently, with no one to check on her. I called the Senior Living Options rep again and told her our concerns. She was quick to respond. The next day we set out to look at several residential homes that usually took in four to five residents. These were homes whose bedrooms were converted for use of the residents. The ones we could afford were either retro 1970s decor or had two people to a room. I wasn't really comfortable with any of them, as I tried to picture my mother with a roommate. After she had lived by herself in a house for twelve years, could she share one room with a stranger? No way. I was discouraged.

The next day the representative called. "I think I found the perfect place for your mom," she said. "A new home has opened up and it will be ready to accept residents in two weeks." I made an appointment to see it the next day.

She was right. Palm Desert Senior Living, a group of neighboring homes, whose backyards were connected into one large area with grass, a pond, and large patio, was perfect. The home where my mother would live had been recently renovated to accommodate four residents, each with their own clean and nicely furnished room. Laurie, the owner, was friendly, as were as the aides I met. After consulting with my sister by telephone, I signed a lease for six months. Now came the hard part. Telling my mother.

Life at Palm Desert Senior Living

Surprisingly, my mother settled into her new room at Palm Desert Senior Living quite easily. We told her she needed to live closer to me for awhile until she was able to walk better. "Just a few months," we told her. We knew she would be staying longer, but we'd have to deal with that later. The important thing was that she was where she needed to be.

After she had lived in rehab for three months in a hospital room shared with a roommate, a quiet area of her own was a welcome change. Her room was small, but pleasingly furnished with a Polynesian bedspread and rattan furniture that reminded me of what you would find in a Hawaiian hotel room. Since she still walked with a hesitant, shuffling step, she probably also appreciated the small living space. The community living room was just outside her door, which kept her connected with what went on in the house. Three other women lived in the house and were about her age. When they all came to eat or watch TV in the community room, she was able to talk with them. She got along very well with the friendly, young caregivers. However, sometimes her socializing got to be too much.

Each night, one of the caregivers stayed in the living room area in case a resident needed help. Mom, night-owl that she was, soon discovered this fact, since her bedroom door opened to the living room, and delayed going to bed. The aides reported that she often stayed awake until two or three o'clock in the morning talking to them. Of course, the next day she was tired and wanted to sleep in. This didn't surprise me. This was typical Mom. She did like to chitchat, and after Daddy died, sometimes when I called late in the morning I often woke her up.

It was a relief to have my mother in residential care. I didn't realize how much time I had spent worrying if she was eating right, burning the house down, remembering to take her pills, or forgetting and taking too many. I also didn't have to drive to Riverside to run errands with her or take her to the doctor. It was now in someone else's hands.

Soon after she moved to PDSL I was scheduled for my breast cancer surgery and chemotherapy treatment. When I told Lori, the owner of PDSL, about my situation, she said I didn't need to worry about Mom, and to just concentrate on myself and my health. I did just that. I had to have two operations—one to remove my breast and the cancer, and the other to remove seven lymph nodes as a precaution. For the next month, visiting nurses came to change my dressings, but after two weeks I felt okay enough to get out of the house and drive. Luckily, my chemotherapy treatments didn't cause the side affects of nausea or loss of appetite. I did lose my hair, though. I would sit in front of the TV at night and pull it out in clumps. I was bald by Christmas. That gave me an excellent excuse to buy a wig which I supplemented with a hat and cap collection.

People react to dire news like cancer differently. It was my decision to accept it and just deal with what ever that entailed. It would be a waste of time to dwell on 'what could happen.'

I would follow doctor's orders and do what needed to be done to combat the cancer, but I would also live the rest of my life as normally as I could which included checking on Mom.

Now, though, when I stopped by to see her, it wasn't a chore but a visit. I usually took her to lunch once a week. Sometimes we went shopping, but not for long periods of time. My mother had always loved to shop, but with her slow gait and inability to make decisions it became a trial. She might take ten minutes to select a box of tissues. I usually either tried to help her make a decision or stood silently by, but sometimes I got impatient, chose it for her, and tossed it in the basket. Then she would get angry, and I would feel awful. Occasionally, I would leave her to wander around the store on her own. This is not a good idea in a large store. If you have ever lost a child in a store, you know what I mean. I spent a few times in Walmart searching up and down the aisles asking salespeople, "Have you seen my mother?"

Mom had lost weight since her operation and her pants had gotten baggy. One day I said, "Mom, your pants are too big for you. We need to buy new ones."

"No, they're fine," she'd reply, pulling up her top to show her pants rolled up at the waist. It wasn't 'fine'. It made them bulky around her middle. Sensing her resistance, I didn't want to argue, so I decided to solve the problem myself. I scoured clothes racks and the internet to find size six-petite polyester pants, which were rare. I became a great fan of the Alfred Dunner section in Penney's and the Blair catalog. Gradually, I managed to replace all her pants with ones that fit.

She was always grateful when I bought her things and would say, "I owe you for that. Don't forget to let me pay you." The first time, when I was honest and told her I had used her ATM card for the purchases, she became upset and wanted the card back. After that, I always agreed to let her pay me, but she never did. If she thought at the time I had generously bought something for her, she'd later forget we had even talked about it.

DMV Wars

When my mother and I went out, I sometimes took money from her checking account through the ATM machine for her to use. I didn't like her to have much money in her purse because I was afraid she would hide it, lose it, or tip the aides that worked at PDSL. If the aides did something extra for her or drove her to the hairdresser, she told me she liked to give them a tip. I tried to explain to her that they were already being paid to help her and might get in trouble if they accepted a tip, but she was unconvinced. Therefore, I kept a tight rein on her money.

I did let her keep her checkbook in her purse which made her feel she still had some control, but that started to present some problems when she wrote a check. Her driver's license had expired and she didn't have another picture ID. If I was with her, I had to show my license before they would accept her check. It was time for her to get a new identification card.

The day we went to the Department of Motor Vehicles I took her to lunch first and then drove to Palm Springs. The Indio DMV was closer, but it was usually more crowded. I was willing to do anything to make this a more pleasant experience. Who was I kidding? The wounds from the missing car were still fresh.

As we walked into the building I noticed ten people in line so I found my mother a seat and stood in line by myself. I soon worked my way up the line, got the number to be called and the necessary paperwork, and returned to my mother to fill it out.

I hadn't even sat down, when she began to complain, "I don't know why I'm here. I don't have a car."

"This is not a driver's license," I explained. "It is an identification card. You need it when you cash checks or to show identification with a picture."

"I should be getting a driver's license, but you kids took my car away. I can drive just fine."

"Mom, you had several accidents. It's safer if you don't drive."

"I haven't had any accidents," she indignantly replied. "You don't know what you're talking about. I passed my last driving test with a perfect score." It was true. At eighty-five she took the written test and passed. The DMV does not require driving skills tests for seniors of her age, which I question. When family members see that an elderly person is a risk on the road, they have no leverage.

"I don't want to argue with you," I said.

"Of course you don't. You know I'm right." As her voice got louder people began to look over at us.

"Okay," I said. "You want to take the driving test, I'll let you use my car. Let's see if you can pass, then."

"No, I don't want to drive your car. I should have my car that your brother stole from me. I should sue him."

"You do what you want," I said. "In the meantime you're going to get an ID card."

"You all want to run my life," she mumbled under her breath.

With that, I began to fill out the paperwork. I would ask her questions about it, but she refused to answer. When I needed to look at her current license she wouldn't let me have her wallet. I finally had to forcibly take it.

When they called our number to go to the desk I went up by myself and explained that my mother was being very contrary and I didn't know how she would act. The girl said she understood and had dealt with older people like that before. I then went back and walked my mother to the counter. The girl was right. She knew just how to talk to my mother and the rest of the process went smoothly.

After that, Mom carried her California identification card in her wallet. Right next to her expired driver's license.

Another Move

My mother moved into PDSL in August, and in November she began to complain.

"I want to go home."

"I've been here long enough."

"I don't like sharing a bathroom."

I was afraid this would happen. The bathroom situation was not working out. It would be difficult for most women to share a bathroom. Three elderly women? It proved next to impossible. When they used the facilities they took a long time and probably had to deal with incontinence, changing their Depends, and who knows what else. And, according to Mom, they did not clean up after themselves. I know I would not want to share a bathroom after having sole use of my own as my mother had.

"Just until Christmas," we had told her, knowing she would have to stay longer than that. After I finished chemotherapy, I would start radiation treatments which would extend into April. Mom had no concern that it would be an inconvenience for me if she went home. I knew it was part of her dementia. Before, she would have worried about me and not objected, but she had become very *self* centered. Her world had shrunk to where she cared about matters that only affected her directly.

When we realized we needed to find another place, one with its own bathroom, I immediately thought of Legend Gardens, the original assisted living facility we had planned to have her stay upon release from rehab. Luckily, when I called, they had an apartment available located close to the dining room, so she would not have far to walk.

We made the move to Legend Gardens right after Christmas. The apartment came unfurnished, so one weekend my husband and I, along with Barb and Roy, drove to Mom's house in Riverside. We loaded the truck with the bed, dresser and dressing table from her guest bedroom, a small sofa and some end tables from the living room, along with family pictures and knickknacks we thought she would like. If we made it feel like "home" we thought it might ease the transition, and she would not be too upset.

Unfortunately, she was extremely upset. When we drove into the parking lot that first day, she refused to get out of the car. We left her sitting there as we all went into her apartment, giving her time to cool down. Finally, I went back out to talk with her, performing the role of conciliator. Over the years, I had learned to remain calm and not emotionally invest myself in the situation.

"I don't want to live here," she ranted. "I want to go to my own house. How would you like it if someone told you where to live? I'm glad your father's not around to see how you're treating me."

He'd probably agree with me, I thought. It was hard for her to give up control. I could hear him say, *See what I had to go though all those years?*

"Mom, I know how it must feel, but you can't live at home right now. I can't drive up there to check on you." I really did feel badly, but this was the way it had to be, and she'd have to accept it.

"I can live fine by myself. If I had my car . . . "

" Just come in and see what it's like. You can't sit out here all day."

When she came into her room and saw that we had brought her furniture from her house she was even angrier and we all felt her wrath.

"You went up to my house and got my things? I'm not going to stay here, I don't know why you did that. You are trying to control my life! First you take my car away and now you are telling me where to live! I'm not going to like it and I'm not going to stay here."

With that she folded her arms and sat on the sofa in a huff. We all tried to tell her it was because we cared about her and wanted her in a safe place, but it fell on deaf ears. She was having none of it.

In anticipation of this, I had called a psychologist, recommended by the placement representative from Senior Living Options, who had experience with senior "transitions" like Mom's. He agreed to meet us the day we were to move her into the apartment.

Soon after her last outburst, the psychologist arrived. He sat down for a visit, my mother's arms still folded in defiance. She gave him the same litany: "I want to go home. My children are trying to control my life. They took away my car and now they are telling me where to live."

It appeared that he was unsuccessful; I know he came to see her long after that day, because I saw his charges listed on her Medicare bills for months. When I asked Mom why he had stopped his visits, she answered, "Oh that guy. He was a joke; all he wanted to do was talk. I told him I didn't want him to come any more."

He must have thought he could make her accept the fact that she could not live alone, and that her children had her best interests at heart and were only trying to help. He didn't know my strong-willed mother like we did.

Venturing Out

Now that Mom was living in a more independent facility, she made her own decisions, some of which we did not agree with. When the aides gave her a choice of whether to eat in the dining room or her room, she chose her room the majority of the time.

While we had pictured her co-mingling with the other residents, she did not participate in any activities and declined to go on any planned group excursions. Some tenants tried to befriend her, greeting her at her door as they passed to the dining room, but she made no effort to reciprocate. I think it was partly shyness and partly stubbornness. She didn't want to be there and made sure she didn't establish new ties. She never did let us put up the family pictures; they belonged *at home*.

Television was her main companion. She liked to watch the news, game shows and women's talk shows, but her favorite was California's Gold with Huell Houser. In each episode he traveled to a different interesting or historic place in California. I often received a call from her to turn to that channel so I could see the place where Huell was that week.

Since she stayed by herself most of the time, I tried to get Mom out of her room as much as possible.

She and I still went out for weekly lunches and errands which she seemed to enjoy. Our conversations mostly focused on the grandchildren, what they had been doing and humorous things they might have said or done or any interesting news she might have seen on television. I often tried to steer her to topics that related to something in her past which made it easier for her to relate to.

If someone were to listen in on our conversation it would sound normal for about ten minutes before Mom might start to repeat herself. Ordering from a restaurant became difficult. She was overwhelmed by so many choices. When I saw she was confused, I acted like I didn't notice, and pointed out items on the menu I knew she'd like. Sometimes she studied the menu for a while and then asked me, "What are you having?" After I answered she'd say, " I'll have that too."

We made sure she attended the great grandchildren's birthday parties, and we included her on most holidays. She watched the fireworks with us on my daughter's front lawn, came for the kids' Easter egg hunt in our back yard, and celebrated Thanksgiving with us. My sister visited her as often as she could, and my niece often arrived with a sleeping bag and stayed with her overnight.

I considered taking her on a drive somewhere, most likely to the beach, because she loved visiting the coastal towns and being next to the ocean. Throughout my childhood we made many trips to the beach which was only an hour and a half from home. This beach excursion didn't seem as wise a plan, though, after an unexpected trip our family took with Mom.

My aunt died and we made plans to attend the funeral. Barb and Roy drove from Yuma and we were all going together, a ninety minute drive. I debated whether Mom should go, but she was close with my father's large family, and this was my father's sister. We would take Mom.

As expected, most of those at the church service and reception afterwards at my cousin's house were aunts, uncles, cousins and their families. Mom appeared to know everyone and was able to make small talk. The mood changed as we were driving home.

When we turned onto the freeway she began to question us. "Where are you going? This is the wrong way. I need to go home."

"Mom," I said, "We're taking you where you live now. It's in Palm Desert, near me."

She began to get hysterical "I don't know what you're talking about. I live in my house in Riverside."

"Your house is still there, but for now you live in Legend Gardens. Remember your apartment?"

"My apartment? I slept at my house last night. I need to get home. To my house."

"We are going to Palm Desert. Let's just see when we get there."

With this, she was quiet for the rest of the trip. When we reached Legend Gardens, she seemed to know where she was. I walked her to her apartment and she didn't say anything more about going home.

I knew then that it would not be a good idea to take her away from what had become familiar; a trip away was confusing and would make her long for her house.

Bad Hair Day

A visit to a hair salon had been a part of my mother's weekly routine for as long as I could remember. I'm sure she shampooed and set her own hair when she was younger, but for the last thirty years she had it cut, set and colored with blond highlights by a stylist. Once she found a hairdresser she liked, she remained loyal for years.

When Mom moved into Palm Desert Senior Living, I knew this would be important to her. I didn't expect it to be a contentious issue. When she first arrived, the aides tried to convince her to go to salons that were nearby. She tried one, didn't like it, then stopped.

"She always has an excuse for not going," the aides reported to me.

I began to drive her to appointments. We'd try one salon, then another, each week going to a different one. We even went to Walmart where the young hairdresser gave her a huge bouffant. While I agreed with Mom that some stylists didn't know how to do her hair the way she liked, for the most part, her hair looked fine. The trouble was, no matter who did her hair, they were not *her hairdresser.*

When I picked her up for her appointment she'd say, "I really want to go to Bonnie. She knows how to do my hair."

"But she's in Riverside and you're here," I'd say.

"No, I think she's moved. She's near me now."

Since her dementia, she had lost her sense of geography and everything seemed closer to her, so Bonnie was just around the corner, not eighty miles away.

Finally, we tried the J.C. Penney salon in the Westfield shopping mall. It was located downstairs near the outside entrance, perfect for me to pull up to the blue handicapped curb and help her out. Sometimes I went on a quick errand, but most of the time I parked the car and stayed.

After going a few times, Mom decided they knew how to do her hair the way she liked it, and after a few weeks she found a favorite hairdresser, Rick. Even though she had found a salon she liked, sometimes she didn't feel like going, and I had to cancel the appointment. Rick was understanding. He told me he lived with his elderly mother which helped explain his good rapport with my mother.

J.C. Penney's

Once Mom found a stylist she liked at Penney's, we grew into a routine. We began with her saying she'd call and make an appointment. She never did. She forgot. So the next day I'd call Penney's and make the appointment with Rick.

Every Tuesday night I called to remind her of the appointment which I set for Wednesday. I also called on Wednesday morning to remind her, but by then she had forgotten so I'd have to tell her to start getting ready. Just to make sure, I called the front desk and asked them to alert her caregivers so they could remind her to dress.

I tried to make the hair appointment for early afternoon so we could have lunch first. A Richie's restaurant was in the mall near Penney's which made it convenient. After dropping Mom off in front of the restaurant with her walker, I'd go park the car, and by the time I arrived at the restaurant she would be just going in the door. When finished with lunch, we made our way over to Penney's. While she was at the salon I had an hour to "kill," so I wandered around Penney's and the mall buying things I didn't need or clothes for the grandchildren which made me feel less guilty than spending on myself. Those hairdressing appointments were expensive for me.

I guess I could have used the time to read a book instead of shop, but it was impossible with my addiction–I'm a shop-aholic. For this I blame my mother. I inherited this gene from her.

From my earliest memories I can remember shopping trips with her. There were no malls; we went downtown to Sears, Penney, and Lerner's. We'd often stop to see my paternal grandmother who worked in a small dress store. My favorite store was F.W. Woolworth. My sister and I would walk up and down the large aisles, a quarter clutched in our hands, looking for something to buy. A visit to look at the small painted turtles and goldfish was always on our list. Occasionally we'd leave with one of the small fish swimming in a plastic bag. Other times we'd settle for a bag of candy. After shopping, we always went to Kustner's Drugstore and sat at the counter. My mother and sister ordered chocolate cokes and I'd order a cherry one (I think I liked the mar-chino cherry that came with it.) In later years, we went out of town to Bullocks, Santa Ana, which included lunch at their restaurant upstairs – a special treat for my sister and me, to be sure.

I had great sympathy for Mom when she became so disabled with arthritis that made it increasingly difficult to walk. Her desire to shop was still there, but it was not as enjoyable as it once was. After her hair appointment she liked to walk around Penney's and look. Every so often she had to sit down and rest. Sometimes she found a low shelf to sit on, but more likely we'd end up sitting in the shoe department.

"You go ahead without me. I'll just wait here," she'd say. Of course, by that time I had been over the whole store while she was at her appointment, so I would wait also.

Usually, she had something she said she needed, like a blouse or nightgown. We would proceed on our "quest" for about an hour trying to find the item she wanted. She'd search through racks of clothes, or when she got tired I'd bring items for her to look at. Then, after we narrowed it down to one or two items she'd say, "You know, I really don't need to buy this today. I'll have to think about it." I should have gotten used to this pattern of shopping, but it seemed each time I had high hopes that she'd actually buy something.

While sitting in the shoe department, I'd try to convince her to buy a pair of comfortable shoes which she really did need. Her feet were curled up with arthritis and I could tell it was painful to walk. Her favorite pair were white, open toed shoes with two wide straps that cut across the top of her foot. They looked stylish, but gave little support. The other pair she liked were white tennis shoes which were hard to keep clean. She'd sometimes oblige me and try on multiple pairs of shoes, but in the end refuse to buy any. Usually the shoe shopper gets frustrated trying on shoes, but the only one who left frustrated was me, wondering why I put myself through the ordeal again, and again.

The few times she did purchase something, she'd forget she was the one who bought it. The next time I saw her she'd say, "Is this your shirt? I found it in my closet."

"Mom you picked it out last time we were at Penney's"

"I did? I wouldn't wear that style. Why don't you take it?"

I Want to Go Home!

What finally convinced us was the bell. My mother had been living at Legend Gardens for seven months. She tried eating in the dining room a couple of times, but still spent most of the time alone in her room.

"There're too many *old* people here," she would say. "I don't like to eat in the dining room. A man that sat across from me one time let food collect on his beard and I lost my appetite. And I don't like people taking food from my plate!"

We were disappointed to find that the aides were not friendly, and many of them had limited English, so they sometimes didn't understand what my mother needed.

Most of her complaints were exaggerated, but what was not an exaggeration was the bell that rang any time, day or night. Every room had a cord, connected to the bell, that could be pulled by a resident who needed help. I am sure it was meant for emergencies, but some residents used it for minor problems, and it would ring several times during the day or night. The bell, mounted on the wall next to the dining room, emitted a very shrill sound and was only a few feet from my mother's door. It rang several times when I was there and it *was* extremely loud.

Another concern–the gate to the outside that was near my mother's apartment. This gate, used by the helpers to come and go from the facility, clanged day and night. The sliding glass door to her bedroom looked out onto a small patio and only a four foot fence separated it from the street; to the right of her patio was the gate. My mother constantly worried that someone would come through the gate, or over the fence, and into her apartment.

Her overriding, continual lament, though, was *to be back in her own house*. I could tell she missed Daddy, and she felt closer to him living at home. One day I came to see her and she began to cry. I sat down on the couch next to her.

"Kathy, is Daddy gone? Did he die? I can't remember."

"Yes," I said. "He's been gone twelve years now."

"How did he die? Why can't I remember that?"

"He had cancer. You helped take care of him. He was in pain at the end and was ready to go."

This was a painful conversation for both of us. I felt sad. How could she forget this important part of her life? This wasn't a short term memory loss. She was mentally capable at the time of his death. Maybe, this was her brain's way of coping with a devastating experience.

The next few times I came to see her she asked more questions. She didn't remember his funeral, and worried about who attended, who came to see her or sent condolences. Fortunately, while gathering her things to bring from Riverside, I thought to take with us the sympathy cards everyone had sent. I brought these to her which seemed to bring comfort. I often noticed them out on the kitchen table where she had been reading them.

Barb and I could see she was not happy, and began to think perhaps we should give her another chance. Even though she previously had rejected every home care agency that sent someone to her house, we thought we could try one more time. Maybe after being away for over a year she would be more amenable.

So we packed up all of her things, rented a U-Haul, and drove back to Riverside with her belongings, my sister and I giving thanks for understanding husbands who we depended upon for heavy lifting.

Mom was home and we felt our caregiver problem was solved. My sister had a friend, Judy, who had recently moved to Riverside and in need of a job. She had enrolled for a few classes at the local community college and agreed to come over every day and check on her, buy groceries and/or cook her meals.

We should have known that was too easy. This arrangement lasted about three weeks and ended badly. Judy had a strong personality, and she and my mother clashed. Mom did not like this woman in her house and resented any help she tried to give. I had never heard my mother curse, but Judy said she received an earful!

What were we going to do? Search for another assisted living facility? Find someone else to help her at home? Of course my mother thought she needed neither one.

Finally, we came up with the idea of asking Mom's next door neighbor, Michele, who had been taking care of my mother's yard while she was gone, watering her plants and making sure everything was okay. They had a friendly relationship. Over the years Michele had come over to borrow things, and Mom drove her to the store on occasion when she still had her car. As my mother grew older and needed more help, Michele bought things she needed when she walked to the store and sometimes dropped by just to talk. After discussing the possibility with Michele, she agreed to check on my mother and help her with errands and light housework; in return, we would pay her every two weeks. This arrangement was also agreeable to my mother. She was happy. Everything seemed to be going well.

The Perfect Solution

My mother was back home where she wanted to be. We were apprehensive, but willing to give it a chance., though her expectations were far from realistic. She thought friends would come to visit, she would be able to fix her own meals and once again go to church services on Sunday. Unfortunately, the true situation was that all of her good friends were either dead or disabled and not able to leave their homes; the knobs were off the stove so she would not burn up the house; and no one from the church would be able to pick her up on Sunday for services–if she could even remember and be ready in time.

Of course, Mom thought her problems would be solved when she had the car back. She promised that if she had her car she would only use it to go to church and run errands like she used to do. That wasn't going to happen. We were not revisiting that scenario. I had always felt better when Mom was on the freeway, anyway. City streets were more dangerous because more decisions were required. If she even managed to get out of the driveway, she would probably have an accident or get lost. She would have to depend on Michele. Michele did not have a car, but we thought she could order the city senior/disabled bus service for her or call a taxi. We also expected her to manage or prepare her meals, as sometimes my mother forgot to eat, or would subsist on unhealthy TV dinners.

Michele took on the responsibility of caring for my mother to the best of her ability. She went to Mom's every morning, got her up and made her bed. She also vacuumed and dusted. We found out she wasn't much of a cook, but she made sure Mom had vegetables, fruit, meat and cheeses on hand so she could fix meals easily. Occasionally, she would bring over meals like hot dogs or hamburgers that she had fixed for her family. She also arranged for taxis to take her to the hair salon every week.

Once a week Michele called and told me how my mother was doing. Most of the time, though, her calls were about her. She wanted to make sure her pay was on its way. I paid her in cash at first, but then when I got busier and not able to visit and hand it to her in person, I wrote checks. A few times when I knew I would be late I had my mother write a check for her.

Even though the family did not go to see Mom as often and she was more or less housebound, my mother seemed happy. She was home! She moved back in September, and by her birthday in June all seemed to be going well. We went to Mom's for her ninety-second birthday. Michele had baked her a cake on her actual birthday, a thoughtful gesture, so we invited her and her husband over for the celebration. Michele gave her a wooden planter for her porch. Two weeks later, when I looked over my mother's bank statement, I saw a problem.

I Should Have Known

I had been taking care of my mother's bills for almost two years. I had all of them on auto pay, and her two incomes, my father's pension, and her Social Security check, were deposited directly into her account. Once she was home, I only had to pay the gardner and Michele. Michele was to give me any receipts for groceries she bought, so I could reimburse her, and my mother still had her checkbook if she wanted to buy them herself or pay the hairdresser. Easy.

Then I stopped receiving her bank statements. With her multiple changes of address the post office sometimes held her mail or sent it into nether-land. I was not concerned. I viewed her statements online. Her balance seemed to stay the same from month to month—until June 19th when I went online to look at her checking account. There were two checks written, one for $250 and the other for $320, both dated four days earlier. They were written to Michele and signed with my mother's name, but not in my mother's handwriting. I didn't care if my mother wrote a check to Michele, but I needed to know what it was for; however, these checks were obviously written by Michele who did not have permission to write any checks. I began reviewing all of Mom's statements dating from when she had moved back home, and printing copies of checks that were suspicious. After about three hours I had copies of twenty checks that totaled $3,700. By then I began to panic.

I called Bank of America and had her account closed. I noticed one check for $200 marked pending and I told them I wanted that one stopped. The bank transferred me to the fraud unit. I explained what had happened and filed a grievance, and they said they would check into it.

Next, I called my sister and brother. My sister agreed to come the following week and we would drive to Riverside and confront Michele. We didn't want to tell my mother, because we were afraid she'd say something to Michele, and we wanted to take her by surprise. Since my brother worked, he could not join us, but when I called him I could tell he thought I was overreacting.

The next Sunday my sister and brother-in-law drove to Palm Desert, and the three of us drove to Mom's Monday morning. My mother thought we had just come for a visit. We decided we needed to act fast before Michele noticed our cars. I had copies of all the checks with me and we sat my mother down at the dining room table and showed them to her. We didn't say anything to her, but her first reaction was disbelief.

"What? This is not my writing. I didn't write these checks."

No sooner had she said this, there was a knock on the door. Michele. She had a small box under her arm overflowing with receipts.

How did she know we were coming? I wondered. It looked like she was prepared to defend herself.

Barb and I looked at each other and rolled our eyes as Michele joined us at the table. I noticed Roy quietly leave the room. He didn't want any part of it.

Let's do this. Let's see how you're going to talk your way out of it, Michele., I said to myself, seething inside.

I showed her the copies of the forged checks. She immediately began to deny that she took the money.

"I would never do that," she said, her voice rising. Why would I do something like that? I know better." She talked very loud and fast.

"You forged these checks. My mother did not write them," I said.

"I cashed them and gave the money to her Your mother said she needed it."

"Where is the money, then? Mom has not gone anywhere to use it."

"She must have hid(sic) the money. She hides it all the time. It's here in the house."

"She wouldn't need any cash, let alone two or three hundred dollars. These were written just last week."

"Some of the checks were for food. See, here are all the receipts," she said, grabbing the receipts from the box and holding them up.

"I know what you say, but we don't believe you. We are going to look into this further."

"I'm telling you I didn't do it. The money is here. She hid it," Michele said, getting up and leaving.

I didn't believe her, and neither did my sister. She was too defensive and obviously lying. We were furious that she had taken advantage of Mom like that.

Mom, who had remained silent the whole time, shook her head and said, "Why would she do something like that? All those years I helped her out when she needed to borrow something, use the phone or go to the store. She was always so friendly. It makes me mad."

OK, we said, Michele said she gave her money, let's find this money. We searched every drawer and cupboard and closet in the house. Of course, we found no money. My sister then took the receipts, and began to add up the grocery costs Michele claimed. My brother-in-law called the lock company and within an hour the locks were changed.

You Can't Stay Here

This time there was no choice and little deliberation. My mother had to move out of the neighborhood. Now. This time she understood. Then came the dilemma. What to do with Mom. After some discussion, my sister and I decided on a rotation. I volunteered to bring Mom home with me for two weeks, she'd then spend another two weeks at my sister's in Yuma. My brother Doug didn't know it yet, but he was going to have his turn after that when my sister and I took our annual vacation at the beach. This would work. I didn't know for how long, but it solved the problem until we could figure out a more permanent solution.

So we helped my mother pack, secured the house, and left. Until then, the longest Mom had ever stayed with us was three days. I didn't look forward to the two weeks ahead, but hoped for the best.

My mother adjusted well, considering the sudden move. She moved into the guest bedroom with its own bathroom, which gave her privacy. She usually slept in, a blessing, because I cherish my quiet mornings to drink my tea and read the paper. By the time she got up, I had her juice and coffee ready. Once she came out of her room, though, the talking began. My mother had always been a talker, but listening to her now for long periods of time was tedious. She would repeat herself often and ask the same questions over and over again.

"Is my house OK? I'm afraid Michele will get in and take my things," she'd say.

"No, Mom, we changed the locks. Everything is safe," I'd answer.

"She could burn down my house."

"I don't think she'd do that. She wants people to think she's done nothing wrong."

Somehow she got it into her head that my husband had a lot of influence within the justice system. As a judge, albeit retired, he couldn't ethically interfere with the investigation. His advice was to let the detectives do their job.

"Has Michele been arrested yet? I thought BJ was going to arrest her," Mom would say.

"No, he is not a police officer. He cannot make an arrest. I am going to turn in a police report and they will take care of it."

"But he's the chief of police, isn't he?"

Even though Mom was driving me crazy with her questions, I felt sorry for her. This was a huge blow. She had trusted Michele and had been betrayed. Because of her, she could not stay in the house that she loved. Though we assured her that her house was okay, we didn't trust Michele, and we certainly didn't want Mom living next door to her.

I could tell it upset Mom. She would go out on our patio and spend time just quietly sitting. She was not her usual, upbeat self.

I certainly didn't tell her about the letter I had received from Bank of America in response to my fraud report. Their answer was that they saw no indication of fraud because the signatures matched the ones they had on file. What? I thought. Michele's big loopy handwriting matched my mother's small precise one? No way! Of course, if they admitted fraud had occurred they would be required to reimburse Mom for all the checks Michele wrote.

I called again and talked to someone in the fraud division, but I got the same answer. I also went to my local Bank of America and had them show me the signature they had on file. They agreed with me, but said there was nothing they could do about it. (i.e.Corporate ruled)

In the meantime, I was busy gathering the materials together to present to the police. I spent hours on the computer researching my mother's bank statements and printing out checks. I felt bad about my neglect, but Michele was clever. The checks were only for small amounts that I wouldn't notice. The forged checks now totaled over $7,000. My sister's analysis of the receipts Michele had saved mainly showed groceries and items bought for her own family, like tortillas and sodas. Barb determined that only $400 could have been spent on my mother. How could she explain the other $6,600?

One of the checks I uncovered had been written to my mother's neighbor, Jack, who lived across the street from my mother. Jack and Patti, his wife, had been friendly with my parents for years. After a visit with us, Mom always remembered to bring them grapefruit from our tree, and they had a key to my parents' house in case of emergency. Even after Patti died of cancer, Jack helped out my mother by bringing her trash cans back up the long driveway after trash day, until he developed back trouble. Patti's daughter, Debbie, dated my brother, Doug, all through high school. Debbie later married, divorced, then moved back in with Patti and her stepfather, Jack, along with her little boy.

When I saw that a check had been cashed by Jack, I thought I had better give him a call. The check was written to him and signed by Michele in my mother's name. I thought it was important that he also know about Michele and what she had done. I was puzzled. Why did Michele write the check to Jack? Did he give her the money? He surely would not have knowingly cashed a forged check, would he? He used to be a police officer.

He answered right away. I first explained to him that my mother would not be home for a while and then proceeded to tell him about the checks Michele had forged.

"I am concerned, because one check was written to you and it is obvious Michele signed it," I said. Expecting understanding, and maybe sympathy, I was taken aback by his reaction.

"Oh, I know all about it. Michele told me. Michele needed the money. She works so hard for your mother, cleans her house, takes care of her yard, does all sorts of things for her," he answered.

What? He knew. And he didn't care? This didn't make sense, I thought.

"But Michele forged my mother's name on the checks. She stole from my mother."

"I believe Michele. She wouldn't do that. She comes over here all the time. We have her taking care of our yard. You know, your mother shouldn't be living alone. You girls just leave her here by herself. You don't know what goes on."

By then I was getting furious. How dare he side with her! "What are you saying? You believe her? She's a thief!" I shouted and slammed down the phone. So much for a good neighbor.

Not only did this phone call tell me how Jack felt, it also solved the mystery of why Michele was ready for us with the box of receipts when we arrived in Riverside. That night I called my brother.

"Doug," I said, "did you happen to tell Debbie about Michele and that we were going to Mom's to confront her?" Doug and Debbie still had a friendly, purely platonic, relationship; he would drop over to see her when visiting my mother, and they would email each other periodically.

"Yeah, why?" he said.

" B e c a u s e," I said slowly, " she told Jack and he told Michele. By the time we got there Monday morning, Michele already knew we were coming and had her alibi all worked out."

I then told him of my conversation with Jack and what he said about Michele. Doug became furious at what Jack had said, and told me what an asshole he was and always had been.

The next day he made it worse. He called Jack and told him off for talking to me like he did.

"I drilled him 'another one,'" he said later.

And the chances for my mother to ever return to her neighborhood looked even dimmer.

Filing the Police Report

I finally finished printing out all the checks that contained Michele's name. I typed up a statement that detailed her relationship with my mother, her employment, and my discovery of the forged checks. I put the statement together with copies of every check that she wrote, along with a list of the check numbers from the pack of checks that I had discovered missing. I was determined to organize everything and present it so the police would have little left to do. What I had to show them proved her guilt. All they had left to do was arrest her. I looked forward to turning in the report so the case could be resolved, and hopefully, Michele would be arrested.

The next Monday morning, I drove to downtown Riverside and arrived at the Riverside Police Department around 10:30. After I found a parking space and entered the building, I proceeded to the front desk. There was no one in line.

"I need to report a fraud and have information for the police," I told the woman at the window.

"You have to wait for an officer on duty who can take your report," she said. "Just take a seat."

The waiting room was small, I thought, for a police department the size of the city of Riverside. The seating wasn't plush, but at least the straight-back chairs that lined the wall had padding. I picked a chair near the end, and sat down. Thankfully, I remembered to bring a book.

I spent the next half hour reading and watching the interesting people enter and leave the building. Most looked like they had been through hard times. Some, I imagined, had committed crimes and were reporting in. Others sounded like mothers or wives checking on a son or husband. At 11:00 I asked at the desk how much longer it would be and she said it could be awhile yet. At 11:30 my stomach started to growl. I went up to the desk. "Is there a restaurant or food court nearby where can get a quick bite?" I asked.

"The Riverside County office building across the street has vending machines and a small cafe," the woman answered, pointing to the right of the door. I gave her my cellphone number in case they were ready for me and left.

With my sandwich in hand and carrying a Pepsi, I made my way back to the police department. I sat outside on a bench eating, waiting for the phone to ring, then wandered back inside and took out my book. Fifty pages later, they called me to the desk. By then it was 12:30.

A young female officer came out and led me through the locked door at the back of the room, and into a small room that contained a table and three chairs. As we sat down, another officer joined us. The interview went just as I expected. I explained what had happened and showed them the evidence I had brought. They took notes and asked me a few questions. Officer Ramos wrote my case number on his card and handed it to me.

"Refer to that number any time you call about the case," he explained. "The case will be turned over to an investigating officer and he'll contact you. If you don't hear anything within a week or two, you can call the number on the card."

I left the building for the drive home, exhausted, but feeling as if a weight had been lifted from my shoulders. It was now their responsibility. I just had to wait for the investigator's call.

Shlepping Mom

Mom stayed with my husband and me for two weeks, and then I drove her to my sister's house in Yuma. Two weeks after that Doug picked her up and took her to his house. We then planned to start over again.

Of course our plan didn't work. Our mother was so confused she didn't remember where she was half the time. It would have to be assisted living, once again. Since I had been through this search already the year before, I knew what each facility offered. I called Senior Living Options and was put in touch with their representative. My sister thought Mom should go to a private home and we looked at a few, but I was not happy with what I found. There was one assisted living facility, Atria, that I had liked the year before, but didn't choose, because it was a little higher in price; however, after some negotiation help from the representative, we were able to secure a room for my mother. Atria assisted living was clean and friendly and had an activity program and beautiful dining room. And it was again close to me.

We took a weekend to move in my mother's mahogany guest room furniture and two living room chairs, one pink and the other avocado green. I then went out shopping. I decided this time to try to make my mother's room look like a well-appointed hotel room. I knew she was like me—not comfortable in rooms that weren't color coordinated and nicely decorated. In Marshall's, I found a beautiful quilt and matching pillows with large pink flowers. Over the internet, I ordered a small table for her kitchen area, and finished with a pale green rug and two artificial floor plants from Kohl's. I hoped this would sell her on the room, like the staging of a house for sale.

She did like her room and soon became used to the routine of the place. She had many options to choose from there, from food to activities; Atria also assigned a resident to talk with her and show her around. She was friendly with the aides and often joked with them about how hard they worked. We had high expectations that she would become part of the community. My mother had other ideas.

You Can't Make Me

My mother needed a doctor's exam and health report before she was admitted to Atria. This is required by all assisted living facilities. Before she entered Palm Desert Senior Living and Legend Gardens she saw a local doctor and, of course, complained about him. I wanted to find a new doctor for her, one that would be a better fit.

I searched the phone book, called the local hospital for referrals and then Googled the names of the doctors to check their credentials and backgrounds. I finally selected a woman doctor who specialized in geriatrics. I crossed my fingers that my mother would like her.

The morning I picked up Mom for her appointment, we had just settled into the car when she began her griping, saying she did not need to see this doctor; her doctor was in Riverside. She didn't want to listen when I explained that we couldn't drive to Riverside; she needed a local doctor. Then she switched tactics. During the whole ten mile trip to the doctor's office, she regaled me with a long list of my incompetencies.

"You don't know anything about doctors."

"You probably just picked somebody out of the yellow pages."

"I worked in a hospital. I know how to find a good doctor."

"I don't want to go to this doctor. He's probably a quack."

The doctor's office was on the outskirts of town near the freeway. When my mother saw where we were going she came up with more excuses.

"Look where this office is. It's not in the city. If this doctor was any good he would have his office in the city, not way out here in the country." She looked at me with raised eyebrows.

" See. You don't know how to choose a doctor."

We entered the waiting room, and I checked her in at the front desk. I returned to sit next to her with the paperwork to fill out, which I ended up doing because she refused and wouldn't even sign her name. When I returned the papers to the receptionist I told her my mother wouldn't sign. "Don't worry." she said, "We'll get it later."

As I sat back down, my mother started up again with complaints. I just ignored her, but people began looking over at us. I think my mother thought she might garner sympathy when they saw this horrible daughter trying to force her mother to see the doctor.

By the time we were taken in, Mom had calmed down, somewhat. I liked the doctor. She looked to be in her forties, and from a Middle Eastern country. She asked Mom questions about her health, and Mom said she was just fine, nothing wrong. When I tried to tell the doctor about her hip operation and pain from arthritis, Mom got upset.

"You don't need to talk for me, Kathy, I'm right here."

"I just thought the doctor should know. I'm trying to help."

Then she turned to the doctor and said, "You know, I work in a hospital."

"Yes, she used to volunteer," I said.

"No, I still work there. I was there just last week," she said with a scoff.

By this time the doctor seemed to understand and asked Mom a few questions to check for memory loss. She then said she was going to prescribe Zoloft, an anti-depressant.

Yes. Something to make her more positive.

As we left the doctor's office for our drive back to Atria, Mom was quiet. *Maybe this will work*, I thought. Hoping for the right answer, I asked "Well, what did you think of the doctor? She seemed nice."

"She's not a real doctor. She isn't in the city. I'll wait and go to my doctor in Riverside."

A Bloody Standoff

The doctor referred my mother for lab work. It is a usual procedure when you see a new doctor. But my mother knew better. It was a simple blood draw, but you would think I was taking her to a coven of vampires.

Her follow-up appointment with the doctor neared, and I knew she needed to have the bloodwork done so the results could be sent to the doctor. Anticipating some resistance, I only told her we were going out to lunch the day I picked her up at Atria. After a few miles, I said "While we're out, we"ll stop by the lab. Your doctor appointment is next week." Not hearing a response, I began to think there would be no problem. Then we pulled into the parking lot of the office building where the medical lab was located.

"Why are we stopping here?" my mother said.

"I told you. You need some blood-work done before your next appointment," I answered.

"You don't know where you're going. You just can't drive up to a place and give them your blood."

"Mom, this is where the lab is. See, here is the paper the doctor gave you," I said showing it to her.

"I don't care. They're not getting my blood. I've never been here before. We don't know these people."

By then I had parked and turned off the engine. It was a hot day, 112 degrees, and it was still morning. I got out and went over to her side of the car.

"C'mon Mom. Let's go in. It won't take that long."

"No, I'm not going in there. You can't trust those people."

I spent the next twenty minutes trying to convince her to get out of the car. Finally I gave up and said, "I'm going to go to the lab and tell them we'll be there in a few minutes."

I went into Lab Corp and told them I was bringing my mother in for a blood draw, but was meeting with resistance. I let them know she had dementia and could be very contrary. They said they understood and to bring her in when I could. There was no one else in the office at that time.

I returned to the car. My mother was still sitting there, sweat pouring off her face.

"OK, Mom," I said. "I can see you are all hot and sweaty. Please get out of the car."

"No. I'm not getting out, " she said with a sneer.

It was at that point I lost my patience. I refused to give in. I called my brother. He was always telling me how he would handle things with her. Let him try.

I soon had him on the phone and explained the situation to him. I handed the phone to Mom. She listened to him talk for awhile, then said, "No. I'm not going to do it. Kathy doesn't even know these people. You don't either. I'm getting tired of you kids telling me what to do. I used to work in a doctor's office and know about doctors and tests. You don't."

After more talk back and forth, I finally took the phone back. "Thanks for trying, " I said.
"I'll keep you posted."

"So you just had to call your brother, didn't you?" Mom said. "He doesn't know anymore than you do."

I left and went back into the lab. "Do you have a wheelchair I could use?" I asked.

They said they didn't, but I could probably borrow one from the doctor's office on the other side of the building. This complex of offices all faced the outside and was connected by a series of sidewalks. I walked to the other side, mostly in the sun, and retrieved a wheelchair.

I didn't know how I was going to get my mother into the chair, but I would try. This would be my final effort. At this point I was tempted to call a taxi and leave her there.

When I came back around the corner to the car I was surprised to see Mom sitting outside on a brick planter. She did not put up much resistance and got into the wheelchair. We finally entered the medical lab. The receptionist and nurse were ready for us.

"I'm not going to do it," my mother said. "You know, you're not real nurses," she continued, as the nurse wheeled her out of the room.

That night I texted my brother my final success, and sat down with a glass of wine to tell my husband the newest "Mom" story.

"Look," I said. "She's even driven me to drink."

Gamma

It was my son Brant's first child and he was excited to show him off. When he and his wife came to see us a few months after the baby was born, he made sure to take him to see my mother at Palm Desert Senior Living where she was staying at the time. I went along.

Of course, Grandma was thrilled to meet the newest member of the family. She got to hold him and remark on what a beautiful baby he was.

"He looks just like his daddy," she said over and over. He *was* a small version of my son, with his dark hair and brown eyes.

" Where do you live now?" Mom asked him.

"We live in Venice, near the beach," my son answered.

" You know, my father used to own some land near there. He had to let it go for taxes during the depression. Now it's part of the LA airport."

"Wow," my son said. "If only he could have saved it."

" Yes, but he was lucky to have a job."

A few minutes later Mom asked," Where do you live now?" and my son responded patiently, "Venice."

The next time she asked the question, he turned to me with a 'what's up' question in his eyes. Brant had not seen his grandmother since her fall and rehabilitation, so he was not prepared for the change in her. In response, I gave a slight shake of my head and waved my hands back and forth, indicating 'let it go.'

When we got back to our house, Brant questioned me. "What's wrong with Gamma? How long has she been this way?'

"She was beginning to have memory problems, but after her fall and operation it's become worse," I answered.

"Geez. I feel so bad for her. Is she going to get better?"

"No. She has dementia, maybe Alzheimer's. She's probably going to get worse."

"That sucks. But at least she knows us, and I'm glad she got to see the baby."

Mom has always had a good relationship with the grandchildren. My two, along with my sister's and brother's children, spent many vacations with her and my dad. She always planned things for them to do and they sometimes took them on their vacations to the beach.

As they became adults they did not visit as often, but would see her on holidays. After she moved to assisted living, and her mental health started to decline, the two granddaughters visited more often and called her at least twice a week. My daughter, who lived near her, was able to see her more. My sister's daughter, Megan, who lived in Arizona tried to come once a month. She would bring her daughter and their sleeping bags and sleep on the floor in her room. They were welcome to stay at my house, but elected to stay there. It wouldn't have been my choice, but she didn't seem to mind

"Gamma likes to have us with her," my niece would say.

Like most families, over the years we have developed traditions. When my daughter became an adult, she and her grandmother started their own tradition. They were both fond of Bloody Marys. On holidays, my daughter would make one for herself and one for her grandmother. It got to be a joke between them. After my dad died we usually celebrated holidays at our house, and the minute Mom came in the door that day she would say, "Okay, where's my Bloody Mary?"

My daughter would have it ready and hand it to her.

While not loud and boisterous, my mother was not above kidding or teasing in her own quiet way. One holiday, when Mom was living at Atria, we were all seated at our dining room table and my daughter was telling a story, when the subject of age came up. "I don't want to grow old," she said. Just then, she remembered my mother sitting across from her. "I didn't mean . . . I wouldn't mind . . . Gamma, I'm glad you're . . . your age."

We were surprised when Mom answered, without pause, "That's okay, Ricki. I'm going to live to be 110, and when I'm 109 you're going to say, *Isn't she dead yet?*"

We all had to laugh.

This affection for Gamma also extended to the great-grandchildren. My niece's teenagers called her to see how she was, and the little ones sent pictures. My young granddaughter was learning to write, and loved creating notes with pictures. When she came over to my house for a visit, she liked to use the free notecards I received from the environmental organizations I contributed to. She always wrote one to Mom. She sometimes included a picture she had drawn. When finished, she'd seal it, write *To Gamma* on the envelope with *I Love You* and lots of hearts, then hand it to me saying, "Will you give this to Gamma when you see her?"

And How Are the Kids?

If there was one thing my mother loved more than anything it was her grandchildren, and this did not abate, even with her memory loss. When her grandchildren grew up and had children of their own and she became physically slower and mentally not as acute, we knew she would not able to do the things with the great-grandchildren that she had been able to do with her grandkids. Sometimes, it was hard for her to realize that.

When she saw my daughter who lived near Atria, she would say," Bring the kids over any time. I can watch them for you."

"We'll see," my daughter would reply tactfully, trying to picture her very active three and five-year-olds alone in the room with her grandmother for even ten minutes.

Mom must have realized her own nightmare, though. One day she and I went out to lunch with my daughter and the two great-grandkids. The lunch went well, the kids were good, if a bit squirmy, which was normal. That must have been on her mind because at ten o'clock the next night I got a phone call.

"Are you coming to pick up the kids?"

Her question did not surprise me. In her confusion, she often thought my grandchildren lived with
me.

"What kids?" I said. "You mean Ricki's?"

"Yes. They're running around the room and up
and down the hall. I've tried to get them to stop.
They've been here all afternoon."

" I will call Ricki," I said, playing along.

" No, Ricki is here too," she replied.

"Let me talk with her," I said.

When my mother turned from the phone and
called for her I knew I had gone too far with this game.

"She must have gone out of the room," my
mother said.

"She probably took them home," I said.

Just then there was a knock on my mother's door
and I heard an aide talking with her.

"Ask her if she has seen any kids in the hallway,"
I said.

I heard her turn away from the phone and ask,
"Have you seen the kids outside in the hall?" and then a
mumbled response from someone, which had to be
some form of "No."

That was my "out."

"Mom, you're going to be okay. I'll talk with
you tomorrow."

And the next day when I called she had no
memory of it.

"How are the kids?" she asked.

"They're fine," I said.

No Easy Answer

Now that we had my mother safely ensconced at Atria, we had to concentrate on how we were going to keep her there. She did have some savings which would keep her for awhile, but all her money was tied up in her house. After calculating what she would save on utilities and groceries by not living at home, along with the cost of her board and care, I estimated she would have just three months before we had to come up with more money. It was easy to see that we either had to rent or sell the house. After discussion, we realized neither my siblings nor I wanted to deal with renters and the problems that could arise, even with a rental service. It became clear that we would have to sell.

Once we made this decision everything moved very quickly. We were surprised when a reasonable offer came in the day after we listed the house. The biggest problem, now, would be what to do with all of Mom's "stuff." She and Daddy were very organized so there wasn't a lot of junk laying around, but the drawers and cupboards were filled as well as the garage. Besides furniture, clothes and linens, were all the kitchen appliances, cookware and dishes, especially the good china and serving ware. Mom also had valuable antique dishes, dolls, and other items that she had inherited. Should we have a garage sale? Do we want to take the time to sort and price everything? What do we do with the things we think are worth a lot?

After deciding time was money, and none of us wanted to do a garage sale, we opted to have an estate sale. Part of what influenced our decision was that the antique dealer who ran the sale had thousands of people on his mailing/email list that would be contacted about our sale. We also asked ourselves what would we do with everything that didn't sell? In an estate sale everything that doesn't sell is reduced in price on the last day and then another dealer comes in and buys what is left at an agreed price and then cleans the house. We would not even have to clean out cupboards. They would take everything out and price it.

Ha! It sounded easy. But we still had to go through everything in the house; open every drawer, take down and look through things on every shelf, and make many, many decisions.

Cleaning out the House

When I entered my mother's house it was the same as I always remembered it. Everything was neatly arranged as if she were receiving company any minute. Her china doll reclined in the child-sized rocker; my dad's army picture, along with the triangle encased flag, stood in its place on the dresser; pictures of my brother, sister and me as babies hung on the walls beside those of grandchildren now grown. But this time it was different. My mother was not there; I was not a guest. I was there as an intruder, someone who was going to search through cupboards and drawers, mess up her neatly kept house, and make decisions about her belongings. It wasn't as if my mother was gone. She was safely away in her assisted living quarters unaware of my deed. I had to keep my feeling of invasion of privacy at bay; this needed to be done.

As I began sorting and handling her possessions my mind drifted back to stories behind each one. It is then I realized I was not only going to get rid of her treasures, but memories attached to them. Not just hers, but mine as well. *These aren't just "things" you are looking at, they are the compilation of the person's life; each item has a story behind it.*

The first room that needed attention was the den and its myriad piles of papers. My mother, being the organized person that she was, had her bank statements and bills carefully rubber-banded by year; however, they stretched way beyond the seven-years-rule required by the IRS. I also found their journals. My mother's contained lists of expenses for each year and month. My Dad wrote in his journal every day telling his daily activities, along with things he bought or places he went. This was a carry over from his time document-ing plant experiments in his work, I'm sure.

Sorting out and organizing took several weeks, not days as we had thought. Sometimes I came by my-self, other times my sister joined me. As we got into the higher bedroom cupboards we found boxes and boxes of greeting cards sent from our families, many with little child signatures and *I love you*s to Mommie and Daddy or Gamma and Papa. These I had to quit reading in order to stop crying and finish what I started. On the shelves in the den were my father's slides and photo-graphs. Unlike my system of "throw 'em in a box, sort 'em later," my father had photo boxes that contained rows and rows of slides and photos orderly arranged and labeled by date and subject.

But it was when I started sorting through the piles of papers my mother had collected from events she had attended over the years that I came face to face with what my mother had been experiencing over the last few years. I began to pull out funeral brochures and obituaries until I had a large stack of close to seventy-five. These each represented the ending of a life, someone who had played a part in my mother's life. In these I saw three women my mother met with each week to play bridge, pot-lucking lunch, laughing and sharing family stories. Her very best friend was here; they talked every week and reminisced about their junior and senior high school years together. Also were my aunts and uncles, friends that died young and neighbors and colleagues. These people were part of my life, though on the periphery. I remembered them clearly and mourned for them anew. It must be hard to lose all your friends. Mom had a few acquaintances she saw or phoned, but no one she could talk to with a history; someone that she could laugh and be honest with. *How lonely it must be to be the last one.*

Packing Up

When we had finally explored every inch of my mother's house we were left with little piles in each room. There were bags filled with papers to throw away, boxes of things we were taking home to store or sell, and items to negotiate.

The biggest problem was: what do you do with the family pictures, ones on the wall, in albums and in boxes? We did not have time to go through them all. We each took the wall pictures of ourselves and our kids and the rest sat. Finally my brother volunteered to take them all, sort them, and scan ones we might want.

I took my pictures home and placed them in the corner of my bedroom where they still sit. I don't want to have pictures of me as a child on my wall. Unfortunately, they will probably stay there until I am gone and my kids will have to decide what to do with them.

Each of us took items that had a special meaning for us or my mother. Among them were her antique doll collection, handcrafted items made by her grandfather who was a wood worker, a china clock bought in New Orleans by my grandmother, handmade quilts and table cloths, and her good china and silver.

We also found some European coins that my father had brought back after the war. The furniture, kitchenware, and linens were all left behind, along with Mom's collection of glass. It was ready for the estate company.

When we signed the contract with the company that was to conduct the sale, the agent advised us not to come to the house after it had been set up for the sale. Of course, I didn't listen. My sister changed her mind about keeping a crocheted bedspread and I drove to the house to retrieve it the day before the sale.

I entered to a house transformed. There were tables set up in each room of the house, and my mother's possessions were strewn across them. As I wandered among the tables I began to get a sick feeling. Everything on the tables had prices, ridiculously low prices. I could hear the estate agent's admonition in my head, "They are priced to sell." Sell, yes. Practically given away, no. I felt like grabbing things and taking them back. I knew what some of these things would sell for in antique stores.

I then asked myself, *Do you want to cart these things around to dealers and try to sell them?* Of course, the answer was *No*. They would probably just sit at home and land on my "to-do' list every year. I went into the bedroom, found the wanted bedspread, and quietly locked and closed the backdoor as I left, knowing that the next time I saw the house it would be bare.

A Bump in the Road

My mother's house was sold. Her belongings also were sold, or in storage, ready to be distributed later. Mom had been living at Atria for five months and hadn't complained about going home. All was well.

Of course, it's when everything seems to be going smoothly that something grabs you, gives you a shake as if to say, *No, no, you've had it too easy. Here's this.*

Only it didn't concern my mother, this time. I began to notice a change soon after the house was empty, before escrow closed. Doug and I were at the house picking up last minute items, when I confided, " I don't feel right. I'm out of balance."

Of course he showed sympathy and tried to understand, but probably thought I was speaking some "new-age hokum."

Over the next weeks, the feeling increased. I became jittery. I couldn't make decisions, and was unmotivated. I tried to fight it, tell myself it would go away. I had to force myself to do ordinary things like fix a meal or wash clothes. There was a large weight on my shoulders. I was uninspired to do things I usually enjoyed. I always looked forward to reading the paper every morning. Now I shunned it. I couldn't endure reading about all the crimes and murders that appeared on its pages. A dark cloud hung over me. I recognized the signs. I had gone through this before.

My seratonin levels had dropped. I was in a state of depression.

I called my doctor. " I need to see you," I said. "My medication isn't working."

At my visit, the doctor confirmed that I was indeed suffering from depression, and prescribed a new medication for me; however, that did not mean I would get better right away. Before starting a new antidepressant, the dosage of the current medication needs to be gradually reduced. Then, the new medication is commenced, the dosage slowly increased until it becomes effective and the symptoms of depression have gone. This could take months.

My condition worsened when I began to decrease the medication. When I was away from the house, and around other people, I could keep myself together, keep my mind at bay. Alone at home, and in the evenings, though, my mind explored the darker side. I felt worthless. I over-reacted to the smallest problem. I cried easily. My brain was betraying me, and I wanted it to stop. Intellectually, I knew I would recover, but emotionally I felt it hopeless.

During the weeks and months that followed, I pushed myself to carry on my usual activities. I also continued to look in on Mom, although less often.

One day when I came for a visit, the director of Atria greeted Mom by name and stopped to talk with her. I noticed as he passed each resident he addressed them in the same way. If any time I needed reassurance that she was in good care, it was then. It was clear that placing her in assisted living was the right decision, not only for her, but for me as well.

Of course, I did finally recover with the help of my medication and my husband and sister who were of great support. When you have been through depression, it makes you have a greater appreciation for life. It also makes you more sensitive to the mentally ill. It is hard when you lose control of your own mind.

A Call for Help

One night at 12:30 a.m.we were awakened by a phone call. My husband answered and turned to me with the phone. "It's for you," he said.

Still groggy from sleep, I hardly had time to speculate, but late night phone calls were rarely good. The last time I dreaded getting a call was when my kids were teens and hadn't arrived home yet. Now they both had families of their own and I wasn't prone to worry. No, it wasn't my kids this time.

"This is Maria, at Atria," the caller said, "I am sorry to bother you, but it's your mother. She's very confused. She just called the sheriff's department and they called me."

It seems she thought she was in the hospital and couldn't reach any nurses so she dialed 911. *Oh no,* I thought. "We have her calmed down now and are checking on her every half hour," Maria said. *Whew. So I don't need to go over there.*

As I handed my husband the phone, I explained to him what had happened.

"Your poor mother. Thank God her last name is different from ours," was his only reply as he fell back to sleep. Even though he meant it as a joke, I understood how law enforcement personnel might have made a connection.

When I went to see her the next day she was fine of course and had no memory of the previous night; however, someone had placed a large sign above her telephone: **FRONT DESK 555-1212**

Patience

Living with or helping an elderly person takes patience. Lots of patience. I thought I was patient. Didn't I live through my children's teenage years? Surely having taught school for thirty-five years would qualify me. But nothing prepared me for what was required to deal with my mother.

Mom had always taken a lot of time to get ready. Before she could leave the house it had to be spotless; no dishes in the sink, no shoes on the floor, or toothpaste left uncapped. Now the time was multiplied tenfold.

If my husband and I had to pick up Mom to go anywhere I'd call two hours in advance and tell her I would be there in an hour. She'd readily assure me she would start to get dressed. An hour before we were to leave I'd call again. She usually had fallen asleep and the call would waken her. Sometimes she didn't remember we were coming. "Yes," she'd say again. "I'll start to get dressed." At this point I'd tell my husband we needed to go early.

When we arrived, my husband, who had the patience of a gnat, usually decided to wait in the common area and read his book. I'd let myself into the room, not knowing what stage of dress my mother was in. Sometimes she had fallen back to sleep. If she had not begun to dress, she'd have trouble deciding what to wear. Often several outfits were strewn on the bed. She'd ask me which outfit would be best. This, from a mother who had easily made decisions for herself and an opinion on everyone else's, was quite a change.

As a person ages their body doesn't move as fast, but when it is complicated by arthritis with which my mother was afflicted, it took forever just to get out of a chair and move to the closet. Putting her feet through two pant legs and easing her slacks over her hips or slipping her curled toes into shoes was an ordeal. It took half an hour to put on makeup that used to be done in ten minutes. It was sad to see my always stylish, "put together" mother just opt for a quick dab of lipstick because it took too much effort to do anything more. This made me become more aware of my own make-up routine and the time it took. I'd think *Twenty more years of this every morning?* I can understand why the elderly often don't care.

After she was dressed I made several attempts to get her to leave. It always took time to find her purse which she had either hidden in the closet or in a drawer. Her keys were usually in the top drawer, but sometimes we had to search for them. Closet doors needed to be closed and curtains pulled. Most times she had to go back in to get tissues for her purse.

Leaving the room, she'd navigate her walker slowly down the hall, apologizing for going so slow. My sister bought her a newer walker with a seat and large wheels that moved faster. She refused to even try it. She also nixed the wheelchair, paid for by Medicare, which would've made it easier for us to travel with her.

"I just can't walk very fast today. I need to get out and walk more," she'd say. She'd say that every time and I always agreed, both in denial that she'd be better tomorrow.

No More Remote

One Sunday we went to Atria to bring Mom a new remote control for her TV. When I visited her the day before, I noticed that her television was not on. This was a concern because she *always* had it on. When I asked her about it she said, "I don't watch it all the time. I have so much to do, I usually don't watch it in the daytime." I then noticed her remote wasn't on the table next to the chair where she usually kept it.

"Where's your remote?" I asked.

"I don't know. I haven't been able to find it," she responded.

Now I understood. So began my search with an *It has to be here somewhere*, under my breath.

I searched the closet, every drawer, under both chairs and the bed. I even looked in her suitcases. No remote. Did it get thrown out? It was a real mystery. When I told Mom I would get a new one for her I got the usual objections.

"Don't bother. I don't want you to take time to do that. I'll be fine without the TV." T h i s   l a s t statement was not true. She didn't go out of her room and couldn't enjoy books anymore. Television was important to her. It was her link with reality.

That's why Sunday afternoon found my husband and I at Radio Shack purchasing a remote with large buttons that would be easy to use, then driving to Atria. While my husband was busy adding batteries and programing the remote I talked with Mom.

"The toilet roll holder fell down and I can't reach it," she told me.

I went in to retrieve it. "You're out of toilet paper too," I said, opening the cabinet door under the sink where I scrounged around looking for some. No toilet paper.

What I did find was her purse. I had never seen it there before. She usually hung it in the closet behind some clothes or in the drawer under her nightgowns. I picked it up. On a hunch I unzipped it. Yes, there, sitting right on top was her remote control. I held it aloft to show my mother what I had found, and then sheepishly went to tell my husband who had just finished programing the remote and was flipping through channels. All I got was an eye roll.

I put the old remote in the top dresser drawer and got ready to leave, but not before I called the front desk. "Room 16 is out of toilet paper. Could you please send some over."

The Cabin

It's interesting what memories my mother wanted to talk about. With her ability to remember present day events weakening, she would revert to the past– her favorite topic being "the cabin." When Mom was a young teen, her parents bought a large three-story cabin in the San Bernardino Mountains. On a clear day she would often look up toward the mountains and say to my sister and me, "You can almost see where the cabin used to be."

Of course as the years went by and the smog drifted into the valley we couldn't even see the mountains. My grandparents sold it long before we were born. It burned down some years later.

That cabin, though, was still very clear in my mother's mind. She could tell you exactly where it was located, right off the road on the way to Lake Arrowhead on a cliff overlooking the valley. She took you through its many rooms upstairs and down, and described the large stone fireplace in the living room. What she most liked to talk about was *who rented* the cabin. You can imagine, being a teen, how excited my mother would have been when Madeline Carroll, a well known movie star the 1930s, rented their cabin for periods of time.

Since Mom was an only child, she usually asked Letha, her best friend, to go along when her family vacationed in the cabin. The two girls had fun looking through the many things Madeline left there, trying on her clothes and spraying her perfume all over themselves. Mom recalled one time Madeline stayed at the cabin with a man. Her parents thought he was her husband, until my grandfather read in the paper that the husband was on safari in Africa. My mother always wondered who "the other man" was. Though such an event from the Hollywood set would not cause much of a stir nowadays, back then it would have been scandalous.

I'm glad my mother had these memories to hold onto; it helped to fill the void of her everyday remembrances. I liked to hear her talk about them, but was often taken aback when she'd say, "I wonder if Daddy ever sold the cabin?" *I think so. He's been gone 47 years*, I'd think to myself.

One day, my mother shared her cabin memory, and I wrote about it in my blog. That evening, the phone rang. It was my mother. She rarely called anymore. After asking how I was she said she had some news.

"My father sold the cabin in the mountains. I talked with my mother last night."

I was so taken aback all I could muster was an "Oh." My mind, though, was reeling. *She couldn't have read what I wrote! She doesn't even have a computer, much less know how to use one. Mom always claimed to have ESP. Could it be . . . . ?*

But my mother went on, "Yes, I'm so glad they sold it. I didn't like them driving up and down that mountain all the time."

I agreed, not wanting to tell her that grandma and grandpa were not of this life. Instead, I led her on a long discussion about the danger of mountain roads.

My mother began to have more of these hallucinatory experiences. At first, I thought she dreamt something, and then believed it really happened, but many times these experiences occurred in the daytime. While before, she wanted to know how my father died, she now often thought he was alive and was in the other room. One time she told me he was mad at her because her clothes took up all the room in the closet and he didn't have room for his. Sometimes when we were ready to go somewhere she'd say, "Too bad Daddy couldn't join us. I guess he has to work."

Mom used to work as a volunteer at Community hospital a couple of times a week, which she loved doing. Every once in a while, she received a card at Atria from the volunteer auxiliary wishing her well. She would treasure the card, and keep it out to read again and again, which probably reinforced the idea she still worked there.

If you asked how she had been, she might say, "I've been busy. I helped at the hospital two days this week." or "You know, the hospital auxiliary called again, and they want me to come back."

Hallucinations are a natural part of dementia. They can also be accompanied by paranoia. Sometimes those affected become very distrustful and blame others for things that happen. At times, they can turn violent. Mom had the milder version. If she didn't remember doing something, in her mind, she did not do it. If she didn't, then, naturally, someone else was to blame.

"Someone used my toothbrush. See it's wet. I think one of the aides or someone they let in the room used it," she would tell me.

I got so tired of hearing this complaint I went to Costco and bought a pack of twenty toothbrushes.

Then she switched to her hairbrush.

"Look at the hairs. Someone has used this." These are the times you need a sense of humor.

ER Torture

It all started with a snake . . . or a would-be snake. One day I was getting ready to run some errands when I got a call from Atria. It was one of the aides.

"Your mother is sitting in the hallway and won't go back in her room. She says there's a snake under the bed. Could you talk to her?"

Knowing it would do no good talking with my mother on the phone I said, "I'll be right over."

My mother has always been deathly afraid of snakes. It didn't help that when we first moved to the desert we lived in a rural area and had our share of them on our property. Once when she and my dad were visiting one came in the house. I found it curled up under the water heater. Though we whispered and thought we removed it quietly, my mother must have guessed what was going on. We were just sitting down to dinner when my mother said, "I hope you got all the snakes out."

"Mom and the Snake" has been a funny family story told over the years. This time, though, the aides weren't laughing.

When I arrived at Atria my mother was still sitting outside her room. "I'm not going in as long as there is a snake in there!" she exclaimed.

I did a full inspection of the room. "I don't see a snake, Mom. I'm sure it left."

I finally convinced her to come back inside, but I could tell she was continuing to have reality problems when she talked about seeing Grandma and Grandpa the night before.

Soon after we returned to the room, Joseph, the Resident Services Director, who was also an RN, came to see how my mother was. I was surprised when he suggested I take her to a walk-in emergency medical clinic for a urinalysis.

"What does this have to do with what just happened?" I asked.

He explained that sometimes elderly patients begin having hallucinations due to an infection. If an infection that starts in the urinary tract gets into the blood stream there could be problems. *My mother hadn't complained of pains, but she did use Depends, which may make her more likely to contract an infection,* I thought.

So over my mother's objections, I called my husband to bring over my power of attorney papers (just in case) along with the book I was reading (I knew how these visits can go.). After my husband arrived, I convinced him to go along, thinking that he could serve as a buffer between my mother and me, since other doctor visits had not gone well for us.

Luckily, upon arrival at the clinic that afternoon, only a few patients were waiting to be seen, so Mom did not have to wait very long. She was given a cup, and with much time and probably difficulty maneuvering due to her walker, was able to give a sample. Mom was told to take a seat, and when the results came back we were taken in to see a doctor.

"There is some blood in her urine and her white blood cell count is up. She needs more tests which I can't do here. I would like her to go to the Emergency Room. I will send some papers with you so they will know what she needs."

Our long afternoon just got longer.

We drove to the ER, and after checking in with the front desk were soon seated in the waiting area near the admitting door. It was then that the badgering started. When my mother is angry she doesn't cuss or yell. She becomes snotty and caustic.

"I don't know why I am here."

"There is nothing wrong with me."

"You're trying to run my life."

"You don't know anything about doctors or hospitals. I've worked with doctors. I know."

I first looked to my husband who tried to placate her but ultimately gave up. The rest of the time he kept his head in a book.

I next moved across the aisle from her, but she kept on. People turned to look. Finally I found a seat across the waiting room as far away from her as possible. It was quiet. I began to read my book.

After about ten minutes Mom was called in to see the doctor. As we were shown into the small room back of the intake desk, we passed several people with white coats who were facing computers. A nurse took my mother's blood pressure and soon one of the white-coated doctors entered the room. The doctor gave an explanation similar to what the other doctor had said. They were going to draw blood to do tests that would determine if there was an infection. Septicemia could be very dangerous.

After my mother was seated in the room next to the "computer room," which held large, comfortable recliners, I went back to sit in the lobby. From the lobby I had a view of my mother sitting in her chair waiting. Soon a young male nurse walked up to her, talked for a few minutes and then left. I knew what had happened.

I left the lobby, passed my mother and entered the "computer room." The young nurse was sitting in front of one of the computers talking with the doctor.

"Are you going to take my mother's blood?" I inquired.

"She told me she didn't want me to do it," he said.

"So," I said, or something like it.

"We can't take her blood if she refuses," he said, with the doctor sitting next to him nodding agreement.

"I thought the tests were important. She doesn't know what she is doing. She isn't capable of reason," I said raising my voice a bit.

"Well, what we can do is call a social worker," the doctor offered. "Maybe she can talk with her."

"Great," I said.

"When the social worker arrives we'll tell her you're waiting in the lobby."

I retreated to the waiting room once again. After about forty minutes the social worker, a large amiable woman, approached me and I had high hopes. She led me back to the same exam room we had been in before, and instructed one of the nurse's assistants to get my mother who was still seated in the chair where they tried to do a blood draw. As I began to explain to the social worker why I needed to talk with her, my mother slowly entered the room with her walker. I still can't grasp what happened next.

"She's crazy," my mother said pointing to me. "I brought her to the hospital and she refuses to have her blood taken."

I didn't need to have taken psychology courses to know this was a classic case of projection. As soon as I had closed my gaping mouth, I began to protest.

Sensing conflict, the social worker asked me to leave so she could talk with my mother alone. Ten minutes later she came up to me in the lobby.

"Have you just been released from a mental hospital? Have you ever been in a mental hospital?" she asked.

"Oh, my God," I answered. "You've got to be kidding. My mother said that? No, I have never been in a mental hospital."

My husband began shaking his bowed head and chuckling to himself.

"This isn't funny," I snapped.

Since Mom's dementia began, she sometimes showed a side of her personality I hadn't recognized before. It made me rethink periods of my childhood, especially my teen years, when she had to convince me to do something. As then, I saw her use manipulation and exaggeration to make her point when confronted. She was a clever woman. But accusing me of being mentally ill? That was going way overboard!

The social worker quickly concluded that I wasn't insane and said, "I didn't think so. We'd better talk." She led me into a private office next to the "computer room" which I had now dubbed Doctor Central.

"Your mother does not want the tests and there is nothing we can do," she began.

"But the doctor says she needs them. Can't you sedate her and do the tests? You can tell my mother is not a reasonable person and can't make decisions for herself." I countered.

"Yes. . ." she said thoughtfully. "Maybe there is something we can do. We can admit her as a 5150 patient. It is usually reserved for a person who is in danger of hurting themselves or others. I'll see what I can do. You can wait in the lobby while I talk with the doctor."

A few minutes later she came out. She told me they would be able to admit her as a 5150 under the Health and Human Services Code. They would sedate her then draw the blood to do the tests. Finally, we were getting somewhere.

" It should take about two hours. "You can call the ER then and find out if she is to be admitted to the hospital, which they will probably do if they find something wrong, or she will be released."

I turned to my husband. "Let's go home," I said. "I'm tired and I could use a drink."

I called at 7:30, two hours later as instructed, and asked about my mother. A nurse came on the line.

"She refuses to have her blood drawn. She is being rather difficult."

"What! Are you looking at her chart?" I said. "She was admitted as a 5150 and needs to be sedated."

"I don't see anything about that," she said. *Good grief! Mom's been just sitting there all this time?* I was more than furious.

"I'm going to call the social worker who talked with me. She can tell you," I said hanging up.

I dialed the social worker and barely began to explain the situation, when our land line rang.

"It's for you," my husband said, "It's the hospital."

He handed me the phone. It was the nurse I had spoken with offering me her apologies, saying she had just come on duty and wasn't aware of the situation. She said they would call when the tests were completed.

We waited. And waited. Finally at nine my husband went to bed.

"Wake me up if you want me to go with you," he offered.

I waited. Decided to have another glass of wine. And waited. Finally, at eleven o'clock they called.

"You can come pick up your mother. She is being released. Her tests were negative."

Should I wake up my husband? I *had* been drinking wine. I decided to just go. At this point I didn't care if the police pulled me over.

When I came into her room, my mother was lying on the bed completely relaxed. She was talking with the nurse. I looked down at her arm. She had big bruises from her wrist to her elbow.

"What happened?" I asked.

"They must have had trouble finding a vein," the nurse answered. "But her tests came out fine."

I looked down on my mother, lying there so vulnerable. I felt terrible. And guilty.

Was I wrong to put her through this? Did my mother really know best?

Hospice?!

After my horrible experience at the ER, I woke up the following day determined to at least see the infamous test results from the blood draw that my mother was forced to undergo. I called the ER and was told I needed to go to the hospital's department of records.

When I arrived at the hospital I was directed to the Office of Records in the basement where a receptionist gave me a paper to fill out and return to her. She looked up my mother's file, then asked, "Do you have your papers of authorization to see her records?"

I took out my power of attorney papers.

"These don't apply to health matters. You need to have the Hippa paper your mother signed which gives you authorization," she said.

I did have this authorization from my mother's doctor in Riverside, which didn't help in this case. In her current frame of mind I couldn't picture Mom signing such a paper for me.

I left empty handed, wondering what to do. Then I thought of her local doctor, Dr. Monroe.

Maybe she could call the hospital and ask them to release the documents to me. I didn't even go to my car; I sat down in the lobby of the hospital and dialed.

When the receptionist was on the line I said, "My mother was in the emergency room last night and had some tests. I would like to have the results released to me. I thought maybe Dr. Monroe or someone could give authorization."

"Just a minute. Let me check," she answered.

Expecting her to refer me to a nurse, I was surprised when the doctor came on the line.

"Yes, this is Dr. Monroe. I was notified that your mother was taken to the emergency room. Atria has called me several times about her."

From her tone of voice it sounded like she was getting tired of receiving calls from Atria. Every time my mother caused a problem, had hallucinated or refused to do something and they called me, they must have also reported to her.

"I'd like to put your mother on hospice," the doctor said.

What?! My mother's not dying I said silently, but replied, "Why do you want to put her on hospice?"

"I want to try a new medication and see if it helps. If you agree, I will have someone call you and they can set up an appointment to talk with you about hospice care."

"OK," I said. "I want to find out more about it before I agree."

I received a phone call that afternoon from the hospice and set an appointment for the next Friday, a day I hoped Barb would be free to join me. I did not want to make a decision like this by myself.

At this point I had no real understanding of what being under "hospice" care meant. I thought volunteers came to your house to assist and help the family at the very end of a person's life, a week or a month before, at the most. I did not realize it was a business that involved many people hired to work as a team.

My sister and I were met that Friday afternoon at Atria by a young Hispanic man who introduced himself as a chaplain. I could just picture how his services were used by the hospice. This sounded serious. He explained to us that a person under hospice care does not necessarily mean they were expected to die soon. A person who qualifies for hospice is someone who needs extra care and not expected to recover from their disease or condition. For the next half hour he explained the process. A hospice nurse would be assigned to my mother and visit her once a week. Hospice aides would help her bathe and assist her in any way needed. There was no cost as any charges would be covered by Medicare.

This was a big decision. My sister and I asked for time to discuss it before we made a commitment.

"What do you think?" I asked.

"I don't know," Barb said. "I don't think she's ready for hospice yet, but she'd get more help."

"I think Dr. Monroe knows how resistant Mom is when she has a doctor's appointment, and I'm sure that she found out about the forced ER blood draw and Mom's behavior. Maybe this is her way to help her get the care she needs so she doesn't have to visit a doctor's office. She can keep tabs on her here."

"I like that it will help Mom, but the idea that all of this will be paid for by Medicare bothers me."

"Me too. As a daughter I like it, but as a taxpayer I don't know if I agree. I think it may be stretching the need for hospice."

Thinking that any extra help for my mother would be beneficial, and understanding we could stop it if we didn't like it, we agreed to the care. Though first she would need to qualify.

That afternoon when my sister and I were visiting with Mom in her room, a large, brusque nurse arrived to interview my mother to see if she qualified.

"How do you feel?" she asked my mother to which she replied, "Fine."

"Who's the president?"

"Obama," my mother said.

"You don't qualify." the nurse said and left.

Well, that takes care of that, I thought.

An hour later I received a call from the nurse confirming that she indeed did not qualify. But an hour later I got another call. "I talked with the doctor. She said to qualify your mother."

Interesting. This seemed to confirm to me why the doctor wanted Mom under hospice care.

The next day I was called by the hospice social worker. She began by saying that she had visited my mother and had enjoyed talking with her. Then she asked what plans we had for her burial/cremation and if we needed help to set up a plan.

"My mother has a plot and it is paid for," I said, a bit peeved. "She is going to be buried with my father."

This was something I did not want to picture just then. I am not one to dwell on the body of a person after they are gone, and therefore, am not a regular grave visitor. My father had been gone for twelve years. His skeletal remains are in the ground, but his essence or 'spirit' is not. His memories are what are important to me and so it will be with my mother.

"My mother is not dying," I said.

"Yes, but it is good to plan ahead. Does your mother have a preplanned service?"

"I don't think we need to discuss this right now," I said.

"All right," she said, finally getting the point. "I just want to be of help."

"What I want," I said, "is to speak to the nurse who will be seeing my mother."

"Oh, she hasn't called you yet? You should hear from her shortly, but I'll check on it."

"I would appreciate that."

"Remember, if you ever have any questions, I am available," she said, hanging up.

That afternoon I received a call from a nurse at the hospice and we set up an appointment to meet the next day at Atria.

When I arrived the next day the nurse wasn't there yet, so I stopped by to see Joseph., the resident director. He was in charge of the aides and residents care, and had to be aware of how each person was doing.

"I'm meeting with the hospice nurse today," I said.

"You know, I still don't think your mother needs hospice at this point," Joseph said. I had told him about it when Dr. Monroe first suggested it, and he had expressed his reservations then.

"It is hard to get my mother to go to the doctor. We think this might be a way for her to get care. If we don't like it we will stop."

"I don't know much about this hospice agency, but if it helps your mother that's good."

By then an aide came to the office door to tell me the nurse had arrived.

The nurse was pleasant enough, but spoke with a heavy accent. She explained how they would visit Mom once or twice a week, help her with bathing and anything else that was of concern. She also showed me the patient directive that would be placed on her door. It said basically that she was not to be resuscitated.

"But I know my mother did not agree to that," I said.

"When a person is under hospice care the relatives can authorize it," she said.

While it bothered me that we were doing this without her consent, I reasoned that at her age, it was the right thing to do.

I got very busy the next week and a half and did not visit my mother. There were no more calls from Atria and I was reassured knowing that the hospice nurse was also checking on her.

The following week, I went to pick up Mom to take her to her hair appointment; we were going to lunch at Richie's restaurant, first. She still wasn't ready when I arrived, which was normal, but what took me by surprise was when we left the room. As we began walking down the hall, Mom took a few steps and then stopped.

"I don't think I can go any farther," she said.

"Shall I get the wheelchair?" I said, expecting an angry reply of, "No, I'm never going to use a wheelchair. I don't need it." Instead she answered calmly, "Yes, I think that would help."

Except for the pain of lifting it in and out of the car trunk, I think I was happier using the wheelchair than she was. Instead of walking slowly three paces behind, or in front of her, we were able to zip into the restaurant and right up to a table. Afterward, I took her on a quick tour around the mall before her appointment. Oh, how free that felt!

My feeling of joy that she had finally agreed to sit in a wheelchair, soon turned to guilt, and then concern.

Overly Sedated?

It was a weekend my sister came to visit that we first noticed how weak my mother's legs had become. She had let me use the wheelchair the week before, but she was still able to walk. I hadn't seen her since then. That Saturday, I was at home catching up on chores and our husbands were playing golf, when I received a phone call from Barb who was at Atria visiting Mom.

"Kathy, can you come help me? Mom has been sitting on the patio with me and I can't get her inside."

"Why doesn't she want to go back in?" I said.

"It's not that she doesn't want to, she can't. She can't get her legs to work."

When I arrived, they were still on the patio. We tried to get her to stand, but each time she tried she collapsed back into her chair. I brought over the wheelchair, and with a lot of maneuvering we managed to pull it to the patio door and hoist her in.

On my way out, I spoke with the nurse and caretakers at Atria and expressed my concerns.

"Could it be the medication she is taking that is making her so weak?" I asked.

They assured me that what she was taking couldn't be the cause.

The week after my sister left, I received two phone calls from Atria. They woke me up one morning at 6 am to tell me Mom had fallen earlier that morning. They called the paramedics, but they found nothing wrong. At eleven o'clock I got the second call; this time they put her in the ambulance and took her to the ER. I immediately left for the hospital.

She had numerous bruises, but after x-rays and an MRI of her head, she was released. It was when they gave me the papers to sign at her release that I noticed one with the list of her medications. I tore it off and stuck it in my purse to check over later.

I got the paper out the next day to see what it said. At the top of the list was *"Haloperidol to be given twice a day, morning and evening."* This must be the Alzheimer's drug the doctor wanted to try, I thought. I googled it. ***drugs.com:*** *"For use in treating schizophrenia. Has been used to treat aggression and agitation in patients with Alzheimer's or dementia, but it can cause serious side effects."* **WebMD**: *"Elderly patients with dementia related psychoses treated with anti-psychotic drugs are at an increased risk of death."*

Oh my gosh. It could be the cause of her falls. And her doctor prescribed this?

I called the hospice the next day, which was Monday, and asked to speak to the nurse assigned to her. I told her my concerns about Mom's medications. Instead of addressing my concerns, she explained that my mother's inability to stand could be a further progression of her dementia.

I wasn't buying it.

Meds

It's hard to know, sometimes, if medication given to help, is worse than the disorder it was prescribed to treat. This is the dilemma I was now facing.

On the Wednesday before Thanksgiving, I made an appointment for my mother to have her hair styled at JC Penney's, and asked my husband to drive us so he could help move the wheelchair in and out of the trunk. I didn't think about moving my mother too.

That morning, when we wheeled her chair to the car, Mom could not even stand up, and my poor husband tried to lift her in. My mother only weighed about ninety-five pounds, but when he attempted to lift her into the car, she held onto the chair, but was so weak she had a hard time pulling herself up. She ended up falling in a heap between the chair and the car. With additional maneuvering and encouragement we finally got her in, although we had to repeat the procedure of lifting her in or out three more times that afternoon. As I had feared, not being able to stand up and walk was not just a temporary condition for my mother.

On Thanksgiving day, my son-in-law offered to help my husband when he picked up Mom at Atria to come to our house. Bless him! Before they arrived I tried to prepare my daughter to understand that her grandmother had physically declined; however, she didn't anticipate what she saw. Mom was slumped over in her wheelchair, lethargic, and was difficult to understand because she spoke in a very soft voice. After greeting her, my daughter pulled me aside and tearfully said, "Poor Gamma. What's happened to her? She's like a different person."

That Friday I called hospice. "I want my mother taken off Haldol. Now. She cannot walk. It all started when she began to take the medication. She also does not have any energy and is groggy."

After insistence on my part, the nurse agreed to talk with the doctor. I then called the med tech at Atria and related what I had told the hospice and said I hoped they were going to change the medication. I asked if she would please call the hospice also.

I got a call back from the nurse in fifteen minutes. The doctor approved Haldol to be reduced in half. That was at least a step in the right direction. You probably can't stop an anti-psychotic medication like Haldol all at once, I thought. I was willing to see how this would affect my mother, hoping her grogginess would go away, and she would have control of her leg muscles once again and be able to walk.

It's Looking Up

Finally, my mother was taken off Haldol completely and I could see a noticeable difference. She was more alert, but still couldn't walk, and I was convinced that her leg weakness and disorientation were caused by the Haldol. An article I read said it can cause symptoms similar to Parkinson's disease. Her inability to walk was a mixed blessing. Before, she refused to use the wheelchair and used the long walk as an excuse to avoid the dining room. When she became wheelchair-bound she no longer had this excuse and she began to let Chico, her favorite aide, wheel her to breakfast. It was also easier when we took her out; we could push her in the wheelchair and were not slowed by her pace.

However, after she stopped taking Haldol some of her contrariness returned and I received another Atria call.

"I just called to tell you your mother is hallucinating and not being cooperative," the medical aid related. "This morning she said she didn't know why she was here, and wanted to leave. She also told the hospice nurse she didn't have to do what she said. We tried to give her a Lorazipam to calm her down, but she refused. Maybe if you came over to see her it might help."

"Don't count on it helping. She doesn't listen to me," I said, laughing.

Whenever they called to report something she did I felt like a parent with a recalcitrant child. I had a ton of things that I needed to do, but agreed to drop by sometime that day.

That afternoon, I brought her a bouquet of artificial daffodils in a white pitcher. It was the time of year her Narcissus would bloom by the front steps of her house. She always picked some and we'd see them in a large ceramic pitcher on her dining table. I thought it might cheer her up and remind her of home.

She loved the flowers, but didn't even remember what happened that morning. She looked fine, great in fact. Most times when I visited she wore a bathrobe, no makeup and her hair was straight and tucked behind her ears. I didn't know who helped her that day, but she was dressed, her face was made up and her hair looked styled, even though it had been four days since she had seen the hairdresser.

As I left Atria I checked the agency sign in log. I saw that the hospice workers visited her twice a week. Though I had serious doubts about their care, I decided to stay with it for awhile longer. It was hard to know if I was doing the right thing.

What Not to Wear

When my mother first moved into Atria organizing her clothes became an obsession for me. Whenever I came to visit I spent time in her closet moving her winter clothes to one end, hanging all her slacks in one section and her tops in another. It seems whoever hung them up did so haphazardly, mixing jackets, tops and pants together. Someone even began to hang up her nightgowns. This was as much a compulsion for me as it had been for Mom. Her closet at home was always very organized.

She didn't like me to touch her clothes, but I'd do it anyway. She'd say, "You don't have to do that. I'll do it later." I knew she wouldn't. Even when she was ambulatory she could hardly stand, much less reach up to hang her clothes on the bar.

Her laundry was washed, dried and folded for her, if she requested. Sometimes when I came she had a huge pile of dirty clothes on the floor of her closet. When I'd ask her about it she would say, "I told them not to do it. I will wash it myself." Many times I would just take her laundry home and wash it.

Other times she had a pile of clean clothes sitting on the top shelf of her closet and I hung them up. "You don't need to do that. I can or have one of the girls do it," my mother would say. Obviously, they weren't doing it.

I began complaining to the caregivers every time I visited. "Someone is not hanging up her clean clothes." I would say, or, "Her dirty clothes are not getting washed."

"I'm not here when her clean clothes come back from the wash." I'd be told by a caregiver. "I'll check on it, though."

"When I try to take your mother's clothes to the laundry she tells me to just leave it. Her daughter will do it," another caregiver said.

For the first year living at Atria when my mother refused to go to the dining room and sat in her bathrobe or "housecoat" all day, it wasn't as important. But after she was confined to her wheelchair and her caregivers took her to the dining room each day, they had to make sure she was dressed to go out.

One day I went into my mother's room in the middle of the summer and she was wearing grey slacks, a coral pajama top with a wild navy, green and white jacket. If she had been aware of what she was wearing Mom would have been embarrassed.

Again I complained to the aides. "My mother has a closet full of beautiful clothes, outfits that go together. Could whoever dresses her please choose ones that look nice and are coordinated?"

After I discovered four pairs of pants and two tops missing from Mom's closet, I began ironing name tags to my mother's clothes. The last time I had ironed name tags was twenty-five years ago when I sent my kids off to camp. I didn't expect to get the clothes back and still wasn't sure if this would deter anyone. A thief probably doesn't care if there's a name tag on it, but I had to try.

Slowly the caregivers began to listen to me. Her clothes were hung up, her laundry was not piled in the closet, and she dressed appropriately. One week when I came to visit she was wearing her favorite black and white skirt with the top that matched. Maybe I was imagining it, but she seemed happier.

"Mom doesn't care how she looks anymore or what she is wearing," Barb would tell me.

"I know. But she *would have* cared, " I always answered.

All her life her appearance was important to her. She wore outfits that were coordinated and stylish. Tops and bottoms matched and bathrobes were for early morning wear. Maybe I was in denial, and clothes were not important anymore, but her dignity still was.

A Search for Justice

When I turned in the police report with the copies of the checks Michele had written, I was sure the detectives appointed to the investigation would start working on it right away. After all, I had gathered the evidence for them, and they would see that the signatures on the checks didn't match. It was a slam dunk case.

Little did I know "how slowly grind the wheels of justice." The day the officers took my report I was told a detective would call me within the next week or two. A week and a half later, I received a phone call from Detective Money, from the fraud division, who said he was assigned to the case. He gave me his phone number.

I waited a month before I called to find out how the case was proceeding. I got his answering machine, "Detective Money is away from his desk or on another call. Please leave a message and he will return your call as soon as possible." I left a message for him to call me back. The next day an officer from Riverside Police Department called and said he was calling for Detective Money. He was a retired officer, but had been called out

142

of retirement to help with the caseload. "There are so many cases, we are backlogged," he said.

I began to call every few weeks, and every time the same officer called in place of Detective Money with the same litany: "He is very busy and will get to it as soon as he can. Try to be patient." When I asked if the detective had even looked at my case or if he knew when I would hear from him, he always replied, "I am not able to give out that information."

At this time, I also called Riverside County Adult Protective Services to report what had happened to my mother. The next week, an investigator from their department came to the house to take down information about what had occurred. When Michele was arrested, in addition to fraud, she would be faced with charges of elder abuse. The investigator told me there were hundreds of cases like my mother's filed every day.

I began to realize that my mother's experience was not unique. Fraud must be common—most of it perpetuated on the vulnerable, older population. That was a sad commentary on our society.

Before he left, the investigator said I would be receiving a call from a social worker to schedule a visit with my mother. This did not happen. Along with the calls to RPD, I began to call the Department of Social Services to inquire about the visit, and was only able to reach their answering machines.

As the weeks became months, my frustration increased. I wanted answers. My mother deserved answers. Why was it taking so long? After six months had passed, I composed a letter to the chief of police:

Chief Diaz:

My mother has lived in Riverside for 82 years. and has resided in her present house for 58 years. Even though she is 94 years old and needs care, she wished to remain at home. We hired her neighbor as caregiver for her last year. It seemed to be going well until last June when I discovered some checks written on her account for large amounts. On further inspection I discovered multiple checks written to the caregiver and signed in my mother's name. It was obvious they were not written by my mother. The caregiver was never given authorization to write checks by my mother or me, who has power of attorney.

I made copies of more than 50 checks and wrote down all the check numbers of ones written by the caregiver. I also wrote a statement that described what had happened and obtained personal information about the caregiver. I gave all of this paperwork to Riverside police officer Ramos when I filed a report last June. I thought it was more than enough evidence to make an arrest and send it to the District Attorney's office.

Since then, I have called the office of Detective Money, who is handling my fraud case, many, many times. I have never spoken with him, but he does have a colleague call and tell me that he still has the case but there are other cases ahead of ours and to be patient. It has been <u>seven</u> months. This is very frustrating. We have had to place my mother in an assisted living facility near me in Palm Desert and sell her house. Meanwhile, the neighbor is continuing to live in her house next door and conduct her life as if she did nothing wrong. Every time I see my mother she asks about the caregiver and if she has been arrested yet.

I know this is not a violent crime, but it is still one that affects others' lives. I would appreciate if you could look into this and let us know what is happening on this case.

Thank you for your consideration.

Kathleen Bjork

Case # P12-090780

I posted the letter via email and also sent a hard copy. I received no response.

My sister and brother were also becoming irritated that the investigation was taking so long. Doug wanted to talk to the detective, so I gave him the phone number. He called and received a call back from the same police officer who had returned my calls.

One week when Doug and Barb came to visit Mom, we decided to drive to Riverside and see if we could talk directly to the investigator. When we arrived and entered the building that held the fraud division I was surprised to find a large lobby devoid of furniture and people. You couldn't hear a sound. This large cold room didn't seem like an atmosphere where you could sit and chat with an officer about your problem. We soon located a small window at the back of the room with a young woman behind the grate, and approached. "We'd like to speak to Detective Money," I said.

Pointing to the wall next to the front door, the receptionist answered, "You have to call him on the phone. The operator will give you the number."

The three of us walked toward the phone, and after some discussion, decided that Doug should call. Maybe a male voice would achieve a better response. We waited, hopefully, while my brother dialed. After listening for awhile, he rolled his eyes, then left a message that we were in the lobby and wished to talk.

"I am away from my desk right now. Please leave a message, and I will return your call as soon as possible," my brother said, mocking the recording.

"We could have gotten that answer at home," I said.

"Yeah, we drove all that way for nothing," said Barb.

After waiting fifteen minutes, we knew no one was coming out to meet us, so we decided to get some lunch and then try the district attorney's office.

We didn't fare any better at the DA's office. We were told that if it was an ongoing case they couldn't talk to us.

A few months later, Detective Money called. *Great. He's finally working on the case,* I thought. After a weak apology and thanks for my patience, he said, "I need a report from your mother's doctor as to her physical and mental health."

"I can send you that," I said, glad to help speed the case along. "I guess you are working on the case now. Have you talked with Michele?"

"I can't discuss the case with you at this time."

"Will you want to interview me or my mother?"

"Not at this time. If you'll get that report to me, I would appreciate it."

I called the doctor the next day and sent the report the following week. I worried that Detective Money would think she could not testify when he read about Mom's dementia; however, I remained hopeful that the other evidence was so strong that it might not matter.

I didn't hear anything for two weeks. Finally I called. When I left my message this time I added, "I only want to speak with Detective Money."

Surprisingly, two days later he called. "I'm sorry to tell you, but we will not be filing your case."

I was in shock. "What do you mean you can't file the case? You have all the evidence. I gave you copies of all the checks, and you can see that my mother's signature is forged."

"The case would be hard to prove. Your mother has dementia. It would be a matter of your mother saying one thing and Michele saying another. The defense would argue that your mother gave her permission to write the checks."

"Okay, my mother has dementia now, but then, when it happened, she *knew* what Michele had done and was angry about it."

"I'm sorry."

"What about all the checks. Did a handwriting expert look at them and see that it was a forgery?"

"I'm sorry I can't give you that information."

"Did you talk to Michele? What did she say?"

"I'm sorry I can't give you that information. Look, I wish I had better news. Fraud takes place a lot with the elderly. A case is hard to prove sometimes, especially when the victim has dementia."

After I hung up the phone, I sat there numb. This wasn't right. This wasn't the result I had expected. If they looked at the evidence anyone could see that Michele was guilty. Maybe I had watched too much television where the criminal who perpetrated the crime was arrested and the victim received the justice they deserved. Then I became upset. I wanted to scream *This isn't fair!* My poor mother, trusting and vulnerable, was betrayed. She would have been able to testify that she would never have let Michele write checks for her, if only she had been asked at the time. But no, they waited a year until her dementia was such that she would not have made a believable witness.

I was so angry I was ready to explode. At the police department. At Detective Money. At Michele, mostly Michele. I didn't care about the money she had stolen, at this point. All I wanted was for her to pay for what she did. I wanted everyone to know that she was a thief. Instead, she would be living in the same house, going on with her life as if nothing had happened. Not having a conscience, she probably justified it in her mind that she was the victim. Meanwhile, my mother was forced to move from a house she loved, one filled with treasured memories, to never return to again.

I finally calmed down enough to call my sister, then my brother. Time to share the anger.

Hair Again

After Mom moved into Atria from the disastrous stay at home, I was once again faced with the hair situation. While I didn't mind taking her to the hairdresser, Atria had a stylist who came to the facility four mornings a week. I thought that would be perfect. She'd only have a walk down the hall to the salon for her weekly appointment. I should have known that was too easy.

One day shortly after she moved in, we passed the salon on our way to her room.

"Mom, look, here is the hair salon. You can get your hair done right here at Atria."

"I don't know," she said. "I like my own hairdresser."

"You could give it a try."

I didn't give up. I suggested it again a few days later.

"She isn't any good," Mom said.

"What do you mean? You haven't even tried her."

"Several ladies here said she wasn't very good." Whether someone said it, she overheard it, imagined it,

150

or made it up as an excuse, I didn't know, but for her that was the end of further discussion.

I continued my drive to Penney's every week. Then she lost control of her legs and had to use her wheelchair. I tried taking her with her wheelchair by myself, once. I managed to hoist it in and out of the trunk and thought I would be able to continue each week, but my back told me otherwise.

After that it became more difficult for her to go to Penney's. Once in a while I had my husband go with me or the Atria van bring her and I'd meet her there. The times I was able to schedule the van, she often wasn't ready or changed her mind. Her hair became straight and stringy. It often hadn't been washed. It was a real struggle to get her in and out of the shower and Mom hated it. I didn't blame the aides; I could imagine how hard it was for them to lift and bathe someone who couldn't stand and was resistant as well.

I thought maybe Mom would tire of her hair looking so awful, and finally agree to go to the on site salon. She didn't seem to mind. I think, though, she rarely looked in a mirror so didn't see how it looked.

Two weeks before Christmas, Doug and his wife were coming for a visit. My mother hadn't seen them for six months, so she was looking forward to it. I thought she would want to look her best so I made a hair appointment for her with Rick at Penney's the Friday before they were to arrive. I also called Atria and arranged to have their van driver transport her to and from her appointment. I had many errands to run that morning and didn't plan to meet the van.

I thought all went as planned, until I spoke with Doug the next day. "I thought Mom was going to get her hair done," he said.

"What!" I said. "It was all set up for Atria to take her."

I had to wait until Monday to call Atria and find out what happened. "We thought you were planning to meet her at the hairdresser's," they said. "We tried to call you."

It was true that I had been out all day buying Christmas gifts. They may have left a message on my phone which I didn't notice, but couldn't have heard anyway in the crowded stores.

"Why would I have to be there?" I asked. "Can't you just wheel her into the salon?"

"We are not allowed to leave anyone in a wheelchair. Someone has to be with her and we do not have staff that can do that."

I did not tell her what I thought of this. What could happen in the salon? Before, when I met her there, I just wheeled her up to the hairdresser's station and she stayed in her wheelchair for the whole appointment. At first I was upset, but later, when I thought about it, I understood–it was a liability issue. However, my poor mother had to go another week with dirty hair.

The next week I called the hairdresser at Atria who she had refused to see. My mother could get mad at me. I didn't care, I wanted her to have her hair fixed for Christmas. I made an appointment for Christmas Eve morning. When we picked her up the next morning to spend the day with us, she still had straight, greasy hair. I found out later that she didn't show up for her appointment.

"My mother's in a *wheelchair*," I said to the hairdresser. "How was she expected to get there?"

It seemed obvious that there was little communication between the hairdresser and the aides who took care of her.

For two years I tried to persuade my mother to have her hair done in the salon at Atria and listened to her constant refusals. I met the Atria driver a few times at Penney's, but trying to work my schedule around the van's became too complicated. Often I set up a time with the salon and the driver, and Mom would cancel. She now had no choice. It had finally come down to: Atria hairdresser or dirty hair.

She refused a few more times and cancelled appointments. Looking at her with her straight, dirty hair was driving me nuts. I didn't give up. I made another appointment. An aide was there to remind her this time and she went. The next day I called her.

"Did you get your hair done, Mom?" I said, waiting for a negative reaction.

"Yes, I did," said my mother. "She's very nice. I like the way she did my hair. Those ladies that said she wasn't any good, don't know what they are talking about."

Yes! I screamed in my head. *Why didn't you listen to me in the first place.*

"I'm glad you like her. We'll have to make an appointment next week for you," I said aloud.

Who called 911?

Mom always had a strong sense of right and wrong, and she was never afraid to let you know it. Her room at Atria had a small patio with only a sidewalk and strip of grass between it and the street. Atria is located in a residential neighborhood, and has its fair share of traffic but we never noticed anyone speeding.

According to my mother, though, the cars that she heard coming down "her" street drove much too fast. When we visited her, she always complained about it. "They use the street like a racetrack. I can hear them put on their brakes. Someday they're going to hit a child."

She also suggested that my husband sit outside and issue tickets. After all, to her he was the chief of police.

One of her cause celebrè did involve the police. Early one evening, a police cruiser pulled up in front of Atria. An officer got out. As the officer entered the facility the director came out to meet her.

"Do you have a resident named Wanda? She called in to the station to say there is a woman in trouble. We have had a hard time determining the problem," the officer said.

The director nodded. "Yes. We know about Wanda. She has done this before. Let's see what it is this time."

Indeed, my mother had had numerous conversations with the 911 operator and several deputies over the course of a couple of hours. After talking with my mother they discovered that she thought a woman down the hall was in trouble and she wanted to help her. When they asked her who she thought was in trouble she said it was May. When the director called me later and related what had happened, I realized the connection Mom had made to the woman. May was the name of her aunt who had died many, many years ago.

Lunch with Mom

I usually tried to see my mother once a week. I felt bad that I couldn't take her out anymore now that she was in a wheelchair, and I pictured her bored, sitting in front of the TV all day. One day I was feeling a little guilty about not seeing her for over a week, so I thought I would surprise her and drop by to have lunch. In the past she had never wanted to go to the dining room for lunch and had them bring it to room, so I thought it would be a treat to go the dining room.

When I went into her room, the television was on, but she wasn't there. This startled me; most times she was sitting in her favorite chair watching TV. I went to the front desk.

"Oh, your mom's in the dining room," Carla, the receptionist, said.

What, I thought, *it's only 11:15 and the dining room doesn't open until 11:30.*

But, sure enough, as I walked in, there she sat with her wheelchair pulled up to a table. What I wasn't expecting, though, was that she was sitting with another woman and as I sat down she introduced us.

"Sylvia," she said, "This is my daughter, Kathy."

My mother has always observed the social courtesies so that did not surprise me. What did, though, was that she remembered Sylvia's name. I wondered how long they had been eating lunch at the same table.

Sylvia, a neatly dressed Asian woman, nodded and murmured hello. My mother told me that Sylvia used to live down the street from my grandparents. Sylvia was from Los Angeles, I later found out, but to my mother that was close enough to connect her to my grandparents' house when they lived in Glendale in the 1930s.

I began to show Mom pictures of the great-grandchildren from my iPhone which she enjoyed, and served to ground her more to reality. After looking at each one, she handed the phone over to Sylvia to look at. Sylvia nodded as she viewed each one.

After a few minutes we were joined by another woman, Ingrid, who said hello to my mother and Sylvia. While Sylvia hardly said a word, Ingrid chattered and seemed to be constantly looking for something in her large purse propped up next to her. She wore a long skirt, necklaces and bangled bracelets, and her hair was in a long braid down her back. If she were younger she could have been thought of as a hippie; now she would be called eccentric.

"Your mother doesn't eat enough," Ingrid said, turning to me.

"I do eat," my mother said.

"Well, you eat like a bird.   She also steals Sylvia's tea."she said.

Both Sylvia and my mother looked at her and didn't say anything.

"I see Sylvia has a teapot. Maybe my mother thinks it's coffee," I said in her defense.

When it came time to order, Sylvia just said, "Soup." My mother couldn't make up her mind until the waitress suggested salad, and Ingrid ordered salad, but complained because they didn't have the salad dressing she liked. After our meals came, Sylvia and my mother ate silently, while Ingrid talked to me. Her sons made her sell her house. She loved her house and didn't want to leave, but she guessed she had to. She couldn't remember where her sons lived, when I asked her. She thought one lived in Palm Springs.

I looked over at my mother saying, "Yes, it is hard to leave a house you've lived in for a long time," but I didn't get a reaction.

Then I noticed my mother, who always ate slowly, was having difficulty. She sat up straight with her back to the chair and shakily brought the spoonful of food to her mouth instead of leaning over, which resulted in half of it spilling down her front.

"Mom, you need to sit closer. You're getting food in your lap." I could see now why some of her clothes were stained and she had so much laundry.

"Yes, you're spilling your food on your clothes," said Ingrid.

My mother reached down and pulled the lettuce leaves off her blouse and continued eating, still not sitting closer.

Sylvia, who hadn't said a word the whole time, had finished her soup. She was soon approached by an aide who asked her if she was ready to go back to her room, and was wheeled away. My mother said she was finished, having eaten only a fourth of her salad. As I began to wheel Mom away another woman walked past the table.

"Aren't you going to speak to me?" my mother said.

"Oh, I didn't see you," the woman answered. "How are you?"

"Fine," she said with a smile.

As I pushed Mom back to her room she said, "I hate to have you do this. I can walk."

"I know," I said, letting her keep up the façade. "Its nice you have friends to sit with."

"Yes," said my mother.

Yes, I thought, even though they didn't have much to talk about, they had companionship. I was going to surprise my mother for lunch, but instead, she surprised me. And her surprise was better.

A Visit to the Dentist

My mother's teeth looked terrible. I knew she had not been brushing them. I hated to think for how long! She complained, "I can't brush my teeth. Someone is using my toothbrush." I thought the problem had been solved when I bought her the large supply of toothbrushes. The next time she complained, I checked for them under the sink. The pack had not even been opened. Maybe, I thought, it is hard for her to brush. It may be too much effort to move her hand up and down.

So I came up with what I thought was the perfect solution. I would buy her an electric toothbrush. I went to Bed, Bath, and Beyond armed with my 20% off coupon. I didn't want to invest too much money into it because I wasn't sure how much she would use it. After looking at all the options, I decided on a simple battery-run model without a stand.

The next day I gave her the toothbrush. She seemed pleased with it and assured me she would use it. After I opened the package and installed the two batteries, I handed it to her. "Just press this button down," I said as we watched it vibrate. She made several valiant attempts to start it, but could not press it hard enough. I needed to take her to a dental hygienist. An understanding one. Soon.

When I called to make the appointment to have her teeth cleaned, I was told that the dentist would have to look at her teeth first to see if there were any problems. I asked if my dentist was available, but he was booked for a month. "We have a new dentist, Dr. Carter. He has earlier openings. I can fit her in in two weeks," the receptionist told me.

"Perfect," I said, thinking Mom would probably like to see a young face.

We agreed on a date, and I decided to wait on the hygienist appointment. One thing at a time, I thought.

The week before her appointment I called Atria to make sure they could take her to and from her appointment. I didn't want to wrench my back lifting the wheelchair, or drop her when I tried to get her in the car. I planned to meet her at the dentist's office.

When the Atria driver wheeled her into the waiting room that day she was confused, as I knew she would be, even though I had called her the day before and told her about the appointment. "Why am I here?" she asked over and over, followed by, "I have my own dentist, why would I come here?" She also informed me that it did feel like she had a cavity in one of her back teeth.

My decision to go with a new dentist for my mother was a good choice. Not only was the dentist young, he was also good looking, friendly, and patient with Mom. After he checked her teeth and they took X-rays, he told us the reason for her "cavity" pain. She had a loose tooth that needed to come out. And it had to be pulled that day. He said he would see to some of his other patients first, and then come back to take it out.

We had to wait about half an hour before the dentist returned. The last time I had been to the dentist with my mother *I* was in the dentist's chair and she sat nearby, so it felt strange to sit there with my mother in a reversal of roles. What was not like the long-ago trip to the dentist, though, was our conversation. By this time Mom knew she was at the dentist's but still was disoriented. She knew that a tooth was to be removed, but mixed up about whose tooth it was.

"Don't you have to get back to work? You don't have time to get your tooth pulled," my mother said, looking at me.

"Mom, it is *your* tooth that has to be pulled. Not mine. Are you trying to get out of it?" I said, trying to use humor to help her save face.

A few minutes later we were talking about my daughter when she said, "How can she have her tooth pulled today when she has to take care of the kids?"

"Now I know you are trying to get out of it," I said. "You are the one with the loose tooth. Can't you feel it in your mouth?"

My mother pushed her tongue to the side of her mouth. "Oh yes, it is loose."

The dentist finally arrived along with a large syringe filled with Novocain. I always wonder about the size of syringe dentists use. You'd think they were going to knock out an elephant, not numb a gum. The dentist had to give my mother five doses before she said she couldn't feel anything, and then it only took two minutes to remove the tooth.

After the nurse packed her gum with gauze and we listened to instructions from the dentist, I went to the front desk and made an appointment for the hygienist to clean her teeth.

This appointment, it turned out, had to be cancelled twice, because of a lockdown at Atria. Though the term *lockdown* sounds like a criminal threat, it was called due to an epidemic of gastrointestinal problems among the residents. Everyone was confined to their rooms for two weeks; residents could not leave, and no one could visit.

Fortunately, the restriction began two days following Mom's appointment, so I was able to stop by to see how she was doing the next day.

"You'll never guess what happened yesterday," she said, when I sat down to talk. "I didn't want to worry you, but I had a loose tooth. But it's OK now. I pulled it out."

She opened her mouth and showed me. The gum was healing nicely.

Happy Birthday

In June my mother turned 96. That morning I went to see her and thought I might stay for lunch. I also had her mail and a small bouquet of flowers. I arrived at Atria at 11:30, and as I walked to the front of the building I noticed someone sitting outside next to the door. To my surprise, it was my mother. Not only had she never done that before, but the temperature outside was close to 107 degrees.

There she sat in her wheelchair, holding a blue and pink helium balloon that said *Happy Birthday!*. Tucked into the side of the chair was a birthday card signed by the staff of Atria. She looked as if she were waiting for someone. It wasn't me. I never told her ahead of time that I was coming, because she never remembered anyway.

"What are you doing out here, Mom?" I asked.

"I'm waiting to go home," she answered.

"What do you mean? Who are you waiting for?"

"What do you think I mean? I'm going to Riverside. A limo is picking me up. There's nothing left for me to do here."

This is where my guilt kicked in. At that moment she looked sad and vulnerable. I knew she missed her home in Riverside, but she didn't know we'd sold her house and that all her belongings were gone or in storage. It would devastate her if she knew. We wanted her to think everything was as she left it so she always had the hope of returning.

"Well, it looks like they celebrated your birthday today," I said pointing to the balloon, trying to bring a more positive tone to the moment.

"Oh, I guess they did give me that. I forgot," she answered.

"Have you eaten lunch yet? Why don't I take you inside so we can eat lunch."

" No, I'm not hungry. I want to sit out here for a while."

After I tried unsuccessfully to convince her to come in, I finally gave up, told her I would return in a few minutes, and entered the lobby. I signed in and greeted Carla at the reception desk.

"She didn't want to come in," I told her, shrugging my shoulders.

" I've tried to get her to come in too, but she said she was waiting for her father to pick her up, then she changed it saying her husband was coming," Carla said.

"Now she is waiting for a limo," I said laughing. " I'm going to her room and be right back."

Since I had to set her mail and flowers in her room anyway, I thought if I gave her a few minutes she would be ready to come in.

When I returned to the lobby Mom was no longer outside. Carla pointed to the dining room. It wasn't hard to find her. She was at her usual table by the door, sitting with her friends Sylvia and Ann. I sat down in the remaining seat.

"So you decided to eat lunch anyway," I said to her, after I said hello to everyone.

"No, I'm not going to eat. They just brought me in here. I'm having cranberry juice."

I was glad that her aides were forcing her to get out of her room. They made sure she came into the dining room every day, whether she was hungry or not. What is more important, it gave her a chance to socialize with the other residents.

Soon, Sylvia left and Mom and I were talking with Ann, when Erika, my daughter, walked in with the two grandchildren. Two young children entering the dining room full of eighty- and ninety-year-olds was like a jolt of electricity. Jayden, the six-year-old, ran up to my mother and gave her a big hug and a present. My mother's eyes lit up.

This was the dose of reality she needed and a perfect birthday gift.

Straight Talk: About Money

What is not talked about, but looms in the background in discussions of elder care, is the price to maintain a "quality of life." Wanting to see that our loved ones have good care at the end of their lives– as they deserve–we are faced every day with decisions to see that this happens. It makes you wonder, though, at the cost.

Few people of my mother's generation had large trusts or savings they could rely on in retirement. Most were hard workers, like my dad, who earned pensions that they thought would carry them through their later years. In postwar America many bought houses and never moved from them; they were proud their mortgage was paid off. Such was the case with my mother. Her house was free and clear, but her assets were all tied up in it. My dad's pension was just enough for her living expenses.

As the one who paid the bills for Mom, I began to see payments in terms of months and years. How long would the money last? How many more years could she live? Of course Mom was oblivious to all this, thankfully. In the past she worried about having enough money. Now she must have thought I had this unending pool of money which paid for her room and board and other expenses. And she still owned her house.

Every month I received a bill in the mail for my mother's lodging, meals and care. When she first moved to Atria it cost $3,300 and it rose a little every few months as her care increased. When she first arrived, she qualified for care level one. This level is for residents who are mostly independent.

Each resident is evaluated by the staff monthly, and given a numerical score depending on how much care they receive. This determines the care level they are assigned. Of course, after she had been there six months they saw that she needed more oversight and help, and she was placed at care level three. This increased the cost $400 which didn't seem too bad. I knew she was not able to make her bed any more, she called for help more often, and asked them to bring her meals to her room. She soon required even more attention when she began to have hallucinatory episodes.

What you don't count on, is that the "doable" starting rate will inevitably increase year after year and month, by month. One day I opened a bill from Atria. My jaw dropped in shock. $7,087! I finally realized they had also charged her retroactively for part of the previous month. In the middle of that month the Haldol had taken affect and she lost use of her legs. She then needed help with almost everything: using the toilet, dressing, getting in and out of bed and being taken to the dining room in her wheelchair, and they charged more for her care, accordingly.

After we sold Mom's house, we put $50,000 into her checking account and the rest into a money market account. With my dad's pension and my mother's small social security allotment, I estimated we could use the checking account money to supplement her assisted living costs for three years before I had to delve into the money market account. Then her care costs rose to over $4,000. I recalculated and determined the checking account money could last for two and a half years.

When her bill jumped to over $5,000, not dipping into the money market account became moot. It was not a question of *if* I would have to draw from it, but *when*. Soon I was writing the last check to Atria from the checking account.

Thankfully, there was another option. When my mother lived at Palm Desert Senior Living and Legend Gardens we applied for veterans benefits for her. My Dad served in the army and deployed to Europe in WWII, and as the surviving spouse of a veteran she qualified for assisted living benefits. She had no assets but her house, and it was exempt. She received those benefits for the year that she lived at the two facilities, but they stopped when she moved back home.

After she moved into Atria and her home had been sold she then had liquid assets so we thought she did not qualify. Barb, who had filled out the paperwork and applied to the Veterans Administration before, tried to recontact them to get some answers, but had difficulty finding someone to talk with about it. Finally, we were given the name of a veterans counselor in Palm Desert who it was said could help us with the application process. My sister and I met with him and he told us if we set up a veteran's annuity account for my mother with her $120,000, a certain amount could be automatically withdrawn every month. This would then qualify her for veterans benefits. The annuity fund was set up and had to wait only a month for approval from the Veteran's administration.

It wasn't long before Mom reached level six, the highest care level, and her bill evened out to $5,400 a month. That came to $64,800 for twelve months, more than most people earn in a year.

According to my new calculations, the annuity would be used up in three years and four months. She could live until ninety-eight before she ran out of money.

For the amount spent on caregiving, a person could live in a four star hotel with room service. It is sad that at the end of our lives so much money is required to sustain us at a time when we are not physically and mentally able to enjoy it.

At times, I considered what it would be like to put my mother on a cruise ship and send her on a world tour. Same cost.

A Dilemma

I can't imagine what went on in my mother's mind; it must have been a constant struggle. The past melded with the present, and it was hard for her to remember what she did two minutes ago, much less the day before.

As her dementia worsened she still knew us and understood what was being said to her, and she could carry on a conversation, but increasingly had difficulty retrieving what she wanted to say. She sometimes used the wrong word; for example, saying *refrigerator* when she meant *television*. Her conversations were filled with events that never happened. She told us she had walked to the store, driven places, and visited with friends and relatives long since gone.

One day I read that one of my mother's good friends had died. Marilyn used to be our neighbor in the days when everyone on the street had kids and the mothers stayed at home. She had a great sense of humor, and she and my mother had some good times together.

Marilyn suffered from Alzheimer's for several years and was in a nursing home. When I talked to Mom about it she wasn't upset. To her, Marilyn was still as vital as she used to be. She told me about what they did together, saying, "I talk to her a couple of times a week."

When someone dies you usually try to console the friend or loved one by telling them to cherish their memories. My mother constructed her own little reality to do this. What a blessing.

I had just returned from a mountain vacation with my husband, daughter and her family when I went to check on Mom to see how she'd been while we were gone. We had stayed in the campground where we usually camped when I was a child, and I brought pictures to share with her. After looking at them she said, "You know, we went there too, the week before you did." I didn't try to correct her; if these made-up memories gave her comfort that was OK.

Mom tried desperately to maintain control and interact like she normally would. I think her strong independent spirit allowed her to keep fighting.

This strong spirit began to get her into trouble, however. Her caretakers all liked my mother, and thought she was a sweet lady, but when she didn't want to do something and felt like she was being forced, she would lash out at whomever was near. At first, when the aides said she hit people, it was hard for me to believe. Then I witnessed it myself one day when my sister tried to cut Mom's hair. She gritted her teeth, said,

"No, I don't want to," and punched my sister in the arm.

One month Atria called to tell me that she was sitting in the front lobby and refused to go back to her room. My mother insisted she had to go outside and wait for her mother who was picking her up. By the time I arrived, Mom was in her room, but not before five different aides had tried to reason with her and were recipients of her wrath. She ultimately gave in when Joseph told her that her mother had called and said she was delayed and would come and get her later.

Mom sometimes didn't remember where she was. One day an aide called me on my cell phone while I was shopping. She said my mother was very agitated and needed to talk with me.

"You need to pick me up," my mother said. "I'm locked in a gas station and I can't get out."

"Mom, you're OK. You are in your room at Atria."

"Where? I don't know what you are talking about? You have to come get me."

"All right. It'll be about 20 minutes. I'm in a store."

"You need to come right now."

I told her I would get there as soon as I could, and arrived about 25 minutes later. Mom was sitting in her chair. She smiled at me as I came in. "Oh. I didn't expect to see you today. How are you?"

"I'm fine, Mom," I said as I sat in the chair next to her. "But how are you? I was worried about you. You said you were in a gas station."

"What? I don't know anything about that."

I was glad she had calmed down. She cut my shopping trip short, but probably saved me some money.

When I visited her a few days later she seemed very subdued. I discovered that her doctor had prescribed Depakote and Celexa through hospice. After I googled Med MD I understood the changes. Celexa is an anti depressant and Depakote is given for people who suffer manic episodes, usually connected with bipolar disorder. I was worried. I talked with my sister and we scheduled a meeting with her hospice nurse. When we expressed our concern that Mom seemed a little lethargic she explained that she was given the medications to calm her down. "We want to help your mother so that she can continue to stay here."

Assisted living facilities cannot accept violent patients. In other words, Mom could not live at Atria if she continued to become agitated and act out by hitting the aides.

No medication: acting out.

Medication: subdued.

What do you do with a recalcitrant mother?

She Needs More Care

The day I dreaded had finally come. My mother had to move. Joseph asked me to come into his office and sign the papers from my mother's three month review and talk about any changes in her care. It was then that he suggested we have a meeting with Vicki, the Executive Director. We met the next morning. They were both in agreement that it was time my mother moved to a place where she could receive more care.

"Your mother needs more care than we can give her," Vicki said. "It isn't just her dementia, it is her physical limitations. She often needs more than one person to help move her,"

This I knew. She had to be helped out of bed and from her chair to the wheelchair. She also needed help dressing and changing her Depends. The problem was, when she had to be moved she could not stand to help and was like dead weight, though she only weighed about 90 pounds. She had fallen more than once, which was probably a liability they also considered.

My mother liked Atria, and I hated to see her forced to adjust to a new room and different surroundings, but I knew it would happen at some point. Fortunately, Atria had another senior living community close by that offered memory care. If their rooms and surroundings were similar to where she was, it would not be as big of an adjustment, and I liked the care she was receiving from Atria. The directors encouraged me to visit this facility and see if I liked it.

"They will be able to give her more help and get her more involved. They have activities that will stimulate her brain," Vicki said, trying to give it a positive spin.

"Stimulate her brain?" I said. "My mother is 96 years old and can't remember anything for more than a minute. Don't you think it's a little late for that?"

I drove to Atria Hacienda, which was close by, and was met by the director of marketing who gave me a tour of the facility's memory care unit. My fears were assuaged. The rooms were not any smaller than Mom's room at Atria, and without a kitchen, they even appeared larger. The common areas, including the dining room, were nicely appointed. I liked what I saw.

Jennifer, the marketing director, showed me the four rooms that were available and told me about a current promotion: if I signed up by the end of the month, which was three days from then, we could have one month free rent. I quickly agreed and we arranged to meet in two days to sign papers. In the meantime the nurse from AH would visit my mother to talk with her to anticipate any problems.

The day before we were to meet, Jennifer called.

"I'm sorry," she said, "but since your mother often needs more than one person to assist her, we cannot accept her into the facility. It is company policy."

I was confused. " I thought one of the reasons for the move to Atria Hacienda was that you could give her more care, including assistance."

I could tell Jennifer felt bad.

"I know, I wish we could help. However, I do have someone who can assist you to help find a place for your mom," she said. She proceeded to give me the number of an agency that helps with placements for seniors.

I had been through this before. I had worked with Senior Living Options so knew the routine. I thanked her and hung up.

I needed time to digest this. What was supposed to be a perfect solution had backfired. Of course, I wasn't given time. The next morning I got a call.

"This is Brad from Senior Living Placements. Jennifer says you need some help to find a place for your mother. I have contacted some in your area and . . ."

A Place for Mom

I finally put a $500 deposit on a place for my mother. It wasn't one I thought I would have chosen, but it felt right.

I received many calls and emails with suggestions from Brad, the Senior Living placement advisor, over the next week, and I spent countless hours looking at places for Mom.

I began with certain criteria in mind. The place needed:

- To be clean, neat and tastefully decorated.
- To have a private room and bath
- Caretakers that were aware of my mother's needs, had experience with dementia patients, and treated them with dignity.
- To show that they were friendly, caring people.
- To have a warm, homey atmosphere.
- A positive feeling about it and a place where I could picture my mother living.

My sister was worried that I would be too concerned about "how a place looked" instead of the people who worked there. I know I am a little compulsive about how a room looks; it needs to be well coordinated with not a lot of knickknacks or frills. My mother's house was always clean and neat and decorated nicely, so I knew she felt the same way I did. Even though she had dementia, I thought she would feel better in surroundings that were more like her home.

Atria had a lot of windows and it felt open and bright. The rooms have large sliding doors which also let in light. Everyone greeted you, and the staff was very friendly, always acknowledging each resident by name. This was the atmosphere I hoped to find again.

I felt a bit like Goldilocks in my search. There was the place that had white walls and floors and hardly any decorations—too cold. And the places that were ethnic or cluttered— too warm.

I finally narrowed it down to two.

Emeritus was a large facility that had a twenty-four bed memory care unit. Residents had private rooms and baths, there were structured activities, and a large activity room and dining room. Every week the residents of the unit baked cookies for the whole resident population. It was nicely furnished and seemed like a caring environment.

Trinity Gardens was built to house up to ten seniors. It felt more like a home. When I arrived, the cook, a friendly older woman, was preparing the day's lunch. The kitchen opened up to the common area and was connected to it by a long pine table where everyone ate. There were windows all along the back which made it bright and warm. Off of the common area were the bedrooms. It had both shared and private rooms. At this time they only had a shared room available.

Which place did I choose?

I chose Trinity Gardens. My mother had to share a room until she could have a private one. I met the lady who was to be her roommate. She did not have dementia, but was limited to a wheelchair because of a stroke. The owner thought they would get along well together.

Why? My mother baking cookies? No way. Trinity Gardens had more of a family atmosphere and I thought that was what she needed at that time in her life.

Uprooted

How do you tell someone they have to move from a place they've come to like, and leave people they've come to know? I couldn't tell the truth which was *your dementia has gotten worse and you need more care, so you don't fit in anymore.*

The night before I planned to move my mother to her new home, I hardly slept. How was she going to react? Would she be sad? Angry like the first time she went to assisted living? Would I have to tell a lie to make her feel better?

I decided I needed to face it head-on first thing in the morning. I arrived at Atria at ten o'clock when I knew she would be finished with breakfast. As I walked in the door she had just been wheeled into the lobby by a caregiver. Her face lit up and I could tell she was happy to see me. As I began to talk myself out of telling Mom, the caregiver gave me an "out."

"We were just going to the activity room," she said. "Your mother wanted to watch them exercise."

"Great," I said. "I need to talk with Joseph anyway."

While they wheeled her toward the activity room I walked up to the reception desk.

"Is Joseph in?" I asked Carla.

"They are all in a director's meeting, but he should be out in a few minutes."

The first person to come into the lobby from the meeting was Vicki, the site director. "How are you today?" she said.

"I'm confused and a bit upset," I said. "I have to tell my mother she has to leave today and I don't know what to say."

"Just tell her she needs two-person assist," she answered.

Yeah, honey, I thought, *I'm sure she will understand that. Never mind how it will affect her.*

Just then Joseph came out.

"What is your usual procedure when a person leaves? Do you announce it? Have some sort of going away party? Or should I just take my mother away quietly without letting her friends know?" I asked.

"It depends," he said." Some leave quietly and others not. There is no real policy."

"What if I bring a cake?" I said.

"We could do it at Happy Hour at four o'clock," Carla piped up.

"Yes, we could do that," Joseph said. "I will tell the activity director."

With that, I left. I had successfully put off telling my mother and I had a mission: order the cake.

My husband, and I arrived at 2:30 to see my mother. He had rented a van to move her furniture into storage and was ready to start, so I could not postpone telling her any longer. When we came into her room she was lying on her bed resting.

I said, "Mom we're here to move you to a new place."

"Why?" she said.

"You need more help." I said.

"Is it here?"

"No, it is a place right around the corner from Atria. It's very nice."

"Oh." was all she replied, and then she lay there and watched as BJ began to move her things from the room. I stayed as long as I could and then left to get the cake.

When I returned with the cake, residents were just beginning to arrive in the activity room. Some had come for Happy Hour and others were ones with whom my mother had become acquainted. My mother was wheeled in shortly thereafter. Soon Ricki came with the two grandchildren.

After some confusion (some thought it was a birthday celebration) those in attendance finally understood that it was because my mother was leaving. As they finished eating their cake people began to come up to Mom to say goodbye and tell her they would miss her. My mother seemed to understand and acknowledge them with "thank yous."

The next morning went surprisingly well. Mom had stayed in a respite room at Atria the night before. When I picked her up she was ready and didn't object when she was helped into my car. Upon arrival at Trinity Gardens the owner and a caregiver came out to help her out of the car. They greeted her warmly and she smiled back.

Settling in to Trinity Gardens

Mom fell again. They said she tried to stand up and fell face forward and hit the end of the bed. Of course this meant another ambulance trip to the emergency room and an MRI of her head. She checked out okay, but needed twenty stitches for the gash in her head. When I saw her a few days later she had several large bruises on her face and looked like she'd been in a fight.

The day Trinity Gardens called to tell me about the fall and trip to the Emergency Room, I was suffering from a bout of vertigo and had been to the ER myself earlier that week and was unable to go. Thankfully, they called hospice, and between the hospice nurse and a caregiver from Trinity Gardens who drove over to be with her, all was well. My reservations about whether to keep my mother on hospice quickly vanished. I was reassured that she would be taken care of in an emergency.

My mother seemed to like Trinity Gardens. After I left her there the first time, I wondered if I had made the right decision. Atria had activity, and residents were moving around, even if it was with their walkers. Here, a circle of recliners or couches was arranged around a large TV screen, and the residents sat there most of the day sleeping or watching television. I soon realized, being with a more active group could not help my mother. Her dementia had made it harder to interact with others and she needed to just sit for most of the day. This is where she was, mentally, at this period of time. I wondered if being around residents who were able to converse with each other easily, might actually have been frustrating for my mother. She tried so desperately to make sense when she talked, but most of the time she didn't.

My worry that my mother would object to sharing a room came to nothing. She did not complain and perhaps didn't even realize that she didn't have her own room. This also served to reinforce to me that Mom was not the same person she was two years, even a year ago, when she would have staunchly refused.

The caregivers at Trinity Gardens were kind and genuinely caring people. When she first moved in everyone remarked, "Your mother is so sweet."

" You haven't seen her when she gets upset and doesn't want to do something," I said.

Two days after she had been there I went for a visit. "You were right," Zairita, one of the caregivers, said. "Now I've seen her other side. She can be feisty."

I laughed. This actually made me feel better. I knew then that the mother I'd known all my life, the one with the strong will and independent spirit, was still in there somewhere and wanted to be heard.

Mission accomplished. I slept much better that night.

The Last Good-bye

Monday morning I had just finished breakfast and was reading the paper when the phone rang. It was Trinity Gardens. I expected my mother had fallen, again, or worse. What I didn't expect was what Zairita, the caregiver, said.

"Your mother is transitioning."

"What?" I answered, "I don't understand."

"Your mother is trying to pass. You might want to come."

I finally "got it," and certainly, I wanted to go. It was now eight o'clock. I ran into the bedroom, threw some foundation on my face, to hell with the rest, and quickly dressed. I pulled out of my driveway at 8:10.

I knew Mom was failing and she had only been at Trinity Gardens three weeks. It was either the fall that was taking its toll or the natural progression of her dementia. Her voice was getting weaker until even with my ear to her mouth I couldn't understand what she was trying to say. It became difficult for her to swallow water, let alone food. They fixed soft food meals for her, but she didn't always feel like eating. Just the week before I was forced to face reality when the director relayed a message to me from the hospice. *They need to know where to send your mother when she dies.*

I had no answer for them. The need to make arrangements was a task I had avoided for too long. Mom already had purchased a plot when Daddy died. She was to be placed on top of him. I had to find a mortuary. After an internet search, I was able to find one in Riverside near our old neighborhood and the cemetery. Arlington Mortuary was very accommodating to my needs. I explained that I did not live in Riverside and wondered if I could take care of arrangements from Palm Desert. They assured me it was no problem and promised to send some materials to look over. I thought I had time.

I arrived at Trinity Gardens at 8:20. I didn't know what to expect. I always pictured getting a phone call and they'd say, "Your mother passed away last night."

Zairita opened the front door

"She's been this way since yesterday," she said. "Hospice should have called you."

"Oh, no," I said. "They didn't. I wish they had."

Zarita showed me into my mother's room and quietly closed the door.

My mother lay in bed. Unlike movie portrayals, she was not quietly sleeping. Her head was tipped back, her breathing loud and heavy. She was struggling. And she had been this way since yesterday! I knew I needed to help her.

"Oh, Mom," I said taking her hand. "Mom, I'm here. It's going to be OK."

For the next few minutes I talked with her, telling her I loved her, we all loved her and she was going to be fine.

"Daddy's waiting for you, and Grandma and Grandpa," I assured her.

I wasn't outright sobbing, but tears began to run down my cheeks. Finally I leaned down and gave her a hug. When I sat up again, she took two more breaths and then stopped. I looked at the clock. 8:35.

I just sat there numb. *I need to tell someone,* I thought, when Zarita walked into the room.

"She's gone," I said.

"That was fast," she said. "You haven't been here that long. She was waiting for you."

"Yes, I think she was," I softly answered, giving my mother's hand a last squeeze then releasing it.

Yesterday was my birthday, I thought. *She almost died on my birthday.* Which made me think further, *she was there to help me come into this world, and I was there to help her leave.*

I sat there for a few minutes, it all feeling surreal, then realized this was exactly what hospice meant. *I needed to call the mortuary.*

The next hour I felt as if I were on remote. I went through the motions of what needed to be done without really thinking about it. I first called the mortuary, but was told I needed to call the coroner first and report the death.

"Isn't hospice there?" they asked.

By the time I went to the office to ask who to call, hospice had arrived. They took over, thank God. They called the coroner and mortuary and had me sign some papers.

I went back into my mother's room and sat down. I looked over at her, but didn't feel the overwhelming grief one would expect. It was more a feeling of sadness, but also of calm and letting go.

Zarita came in. "Maybe you'd like to start packing up your mother's things," she said.
I began to lift the things out of the closet when she came back with large Hefty trash bags.

The hospice nurse came in. "The mortuary said they would be here in an hour and a half."

"I'd like to be here when they come," I said.

First I called my husband at work, and then my sister and daughter who both insisted that someone be with me.

"No, I told them both. I'm fine. I need to be alone for awhile."

So after I had finished packing I sat quietly in a chair in the room and waited.

While some people would be breaking down at this point, I was not surprised at my reaction. Mom was ninety-six. She'd led a long, good life. At the end she was not the same person I had grown up with. Over the years as I watched her struggle with her dementia, I think I had mourned for her a little every day.

I knew I would cry for her and miss her terribly in the next few days and years to come, but I realized I now had the freedom to remember all the times we had together, not just the last six years of her dementia which were filled with worry and concern.

Mom, we've been on a helluva journey together, I thought glancing over at her body. She hated the idea of needing help and apologized and felt badly that she had to depend on me, but she also had given me a hard time, sometimes, when I tried to do so. While it was happening I felt compassion, but certainly didn't see it in a positive light. In retrospect, I can.

Mom was fiercely independent. She was never one to feel sorry for herself; wasn't a complainer. I admire her for this. And her spirit. She was a fighter who fought her dementia all the way to the end.

At 12:30 the mortuary arrived to drive her back home to Riverside, and I left the room after signing the necessary papers.

Zarita met me at the door and I was given a big hug.

"Your mother's roommate, Rocio, wanted me to tell you she is sorry. She prayed for your mother," she said.

"Oh, I'll have to thank her," I said.

I walked over to Rocio who was sitting in a chair in front of the TV where she must have been all morning to give me privacy.

"I am sorry you lost your mother," she whispered. She was a frail little woman who reminded me of my mother. "I prayed for her all night. I could hear her breathing so hard; I knew, and I prayed for her."

"Thank you," I said. "I'm sure she heard your prayers." I reached down and gave her a hug.

"You were a good daughter. I saw when you came to see her."

"You have a nice family, too. I saw the pictures of them on your dresser. One of them is a wedding picture."

"Yes, that's my granddaughter."

"It's all about family, isn't it?"

"Yes it is," she said, giving a little smile.

"I wish my mother had been here longer so you could have gotten to know her."

"Yes. She was a nice lady."

"She was. But she could be feisty too." Seeing her reaction to my comment I added, "I'll bet you were feisty."

"I still am," she answered with a twinkle in her eye.

Epilogue

Seven months had passed since my mother's death, when I drove into my old neighborhood and slowly passed by her house. It had changed. I had high hopes for the young couple that bought it two years ago. They said they loved it, but why did they pull out every tree and shrub to leave it bare? Gone were the trees my father had planted with care, along with the climbing coral rose bush my mother loved that grew beside the back door. The narcissus weren't in bloom as they usually were that time of year, and the front door was painted bright yellow, which my mother would have hated. The house had moved on, as had I.

Next door, Michele and her husband were planting bushes in the front next to their driveway. Anger flared up in me once again upon seeing her. *She continued to live in the same house next to my mother's as if nothing had happened. My mother, forced from her house, was now dead.* I was tempted to get out of the car and confront her. Sound reason held me back. I couldn't trust myself, and it wasn't worth it. It would spoil a beautiful day, and I would probably end up arrested for assault.

I glanced across the street at Jack's house. Jack was dead now, too, but Debbie, my brother's old girlfriend, still lived there. I wondered if she was still friendly with Michele, but I shouldn't care. They were not part of my life now. What I carried with me were the memories of this street in the seven years I lived there from twelve to nineteen, and the happy occasions when I visited Mom and Dad over the years that followed.

I sped up, and left the neighborhood behind. Five minutes later I was at Trader Joe's buying roses.

Driving back the way I had come, I pulled into the cemetery, followed the road to the top and parked next to the hill. I took out the pink roses I had bought at Trader Joe's, along with a bottle of water, scissors, and a spade.

I angled myself toward the small tree that grew a few feet from the curb to orient myself, and tried to remember how far over the grave was located. We had picked this spot for Daddy. It was just a few feet away from the hill that he loved. The hill was perched at the edge of our neighborhood with the cemetery on the opposite side. It was part of our childhood playground. We loved to climb the hill, build forts, and shimmy down rock faces as if they were slides. The grandchildren came to love that hill, too, as their Papa took them there when they came to visit.

After I located the gravesite, I knelt down to cut the flower stems, pulled the grass away from the metal container and filled it with the bottled water. I placed the blooms inside and stood up, looking down at my parents' marker. "Happy birthday, Mom," I whispered, and took a picture with my iPhone, which I would send to my brother and sister.

Last Fall, we stood at this graveside to say good-bye to her. About fifty people attended the outdoor service, mostly my cousins from my father's large family. Only two aunts and an uncle were left from my parents' generation. No friends came; Mom had been the last to go. Chris, the minister, gave a speech and said a prayer. He related the story about his experience with Mom when she fell and he took her to the hospital. It made everyone smile.

When I got up to speak, I was still suffering from vertigo, and when I leaned on the casket situated on the bier, it began to wobble. I could picture the casket opening and my mother spilling out onto the ground. If the mortuary employee hadn't been there to steady it, I think the casket would have fallen.

After the service, we invited everyone to El Torito for food and refreshments. And Margaritas. Mom wouldn't have liked a sad affair, and it was a time to remember family and happy times when my grandma, my parents, and aunts and uncles were still alive.

I remained at the gravesite thinking about my parents. I missed them, but know their bodies could not have sustained them. Often, I see things that remind me of them. Seeing a man taking a walk wearing a straw sun-hat like Daddy used to wear. Hearing something funny the grandchildren said makes me want to call Mom and tell her. I know she would have laughed. Memories like these keep them close.

After slipping my phone into my pocket, I began my descent down the cemetery slope, trying to not step on grave stones. I'd always had the idea that if I stepped on one, it would be disrespecting the person below.

Walking in the cemetery, avoiding the markers, flashed me back to my childhood. Sometimes, my sister and I would hike down from the hill and walk along reading the headstones; in one section pictures were inset into the stone, and we would think about the people portrayed in them. Many of them were babies or small children. We would always finish our tour by stopping by the trash dump where they threw all the flowers that had been on the graves. We'd pick out the ones that were still fresh and bring them home.

Little did we think, back then as thirteen- and fourteen-year olds, that this cemetery would have a personal meaning. Life was an adventure, glowing with possibilities. We had not yet gripped the finality of death.

I turned when I heard crying. Earlier, another car had pulled up and a woman had made her way to a gravesite ten rows over from me. Now she was sobbing uncontrollably and calling out a name I couldn't understand. I turned away, wanting to give her privacy. In the other direction, two young women had spread out a blanket next to a grave and were having a picnic. *We're neighbors now, in grief,* I thought.

Continuing my trek, I passed the grave of Mom's best friend, who she had known since junior high. They had purposely gotten ones close to each other. Ten more rows down I began walking back and forth, reading the markers, until I finally found them. Grandma and Grandpa. I felt a twinge of guilt; I hadn't brought flowers for them. I read the grave marker, Grandpa: born 1878, died 1966, then Grandma: born 1888, died 1961. Poor Grandma. My thoughts returned to the last months of her life and what she had to go through. Thankfully, we now understand more about dementia and how to care for those inflicted.

I'm sorry, Grandma. I love you.

I then turned and started back up the hill to stop by my parents' grave before going home thinking, *They weren't there for me to visit, but they'd leave with me. I always had them tucked inside my brain to pull out whenever I wished.*

Acknowledgements

First, I give thanks to all the readers of my blog who encouraged me to turn it into a book. The task wasn't as easy as it sounds, so I am grateful for the help of Linda Carlson, Judy Thompson and Nancy Ako who helped me bring it to life. I especially give a shout out to Nancy, a master of punctuation− from the comma to colon, and period to ellipsis. I also thank my editor, Kathryn Jordan, and friend and fellow writer, Melody Fleming, for their advice and support. Much love and appreciation goes to my family (yes, all of you) who traveled this journey with me.

Finally, I am extremely grateful to my brother and sister, Doug Drake and Barbara Cavanaugh, who shared in the hard decisions and had faith in me to make the easier ones.

RESOURCES

What Does the Future Hold?

My grandmother was admitted to Patton in 1961. At that time nursing homes would not accept patients who were violent or appeared mentally ill. Hospitals like Patton were filled with patients, like my grandmother, who suffered from Alzheimer's or dementia that manifested itself like a mental illness. Fortunately, there are more options now, as people are realizing the affects of these conditions on the senior population. At-home care, assisted living and special Alzheimer units, staffed with nurses and aides that have the skills to treat patients like my grandmother, are more abundant.

My father's pension, along with her small savings and help from the VA, enabled my mother to spend her last years in an assisted living facility. However, as more of our citizens are living longer, the economy continues to lag, and there is a push to reduce pensions, these options will be out of reach for many seniors. With lack of resources, the responsibility will fall to the family to take on the care of their loved one at home. Hopefully, solutions will be found to lighten the burden of care.

Fortunately, over the last few decades, many organizations have formed to raise awareness and educate people about dementia and Alzheimer Disease

It has has become a world-wide concern. In addition to informing people about the disease, these groups also offer support and helpful advice to caregivers because they understand the the physical and mental toll it takes on them as well.

Research

There is no cure for Alzheimers and most other types of dementia, but scientists have made great strides in brain study and have discovered its causes. Hopefully, there will be a breakthrough in the not too distant future.
These are a few of the sites that provide up-to-date information on progress that is being made in this area.

www.alzheimers.net

www.patients.aan.com American Academy of Neurology- Has a list of studies

www.alzdiscovery.org Their focus is on accelerating the discovery of drugs to help Alzheimer Disease.

www.ninds.nih.gov National Institute of Neurological Disorders and Stroke

2017 White Papers: *Memory Your Annual Guide to Alzheimer's disease and dementia* by Peter Rabins, M.D., M.P.H. published by Scientific American $19.99
Good overview and with the latest research.
order online: HealthAfter50.com/store

Help for Caregivers and Family

Anyone who has access to the internet can find a plethora of information on dementia and helpful advice for caregivers. These are ones I found most helpful.

www.alz.org   Alzheimers Organization

www.nia.nih.gov National Institute on Aging

www.alzfdn.org Alzheimer Foundation-good caregiving tips

www.facebook.com/aplaceformom You do not have to use their services to subscribe to their newsletters. You can sign up on this site. Highly recommended.

www.eldercare.gov Has a list of eldercare agencies by state and region.

www.n4a.org National Association of Area Agencies on Aging-lists agencies by county

www.longtermcare.gov   Explains the Older Americans Act and available resources

www.caring.com Lists dementia/caregiver support groups by area.

www.helpguide.org   Good description of the stages of dementia.

www.agingcare.com Great question and answer community.

www.dementiasociety.org

www.medlineplus.gov National Institute of Health-is the world's largest medical library.

www.lbda.org Lewy body Dementia Association

www.alz.co.uk Alzheimer Disease International-worth looking at-it shows the prevelance of agencies in countries around the world that are working to help combat dementia.

How to Care for Aging Parents 3rd Edition by Virginia Morris Workman Publishing, NY
at Amazon .com a good resource for advice for helping all elderly parents, not only ones with dementia and is currently selling at a reduced price of $8.38